TESTIMONIALS

"This book has been expertly written in terms of readability, unique outlook and charming style. The author engages the reader from the beginning, explaining the progression of Alzheimer's disease while sharing from her own personal experience. This is a heart rending story and one I hope to never go through but it is also a story of courage and coping and I'm sure that anyone facing a similar situation will find the book tremendously helpful.

"Navigating Alzheimer's" will be extremely helpful for friends or family who may know of similar situations but are not sure how to respond to the sufferer or primary care giver. The author's needs and suggestions are communicated in such a way that there is no need to fear being involved with this kind of situation. The suggestions are practical and real and give the reader confidence to step in and help wherever there is a need."

Louise D. , Proofreader

"*Navigating Alzheimer's*" is easy, in fact, enjoyable to read. It tells the truth, but retains that essential ingredient in life - a sense of humour. I believe it is particularly useful for Alzheimer's carers and may offer valuable insights for their medical professionals.

Immediate and extended family and friends will also benefit enormously from the author's experience and understanding of warning signs, diagnosis, younger onset and the continuous progression of Alzheimer's and its impact on the family.

This is a powerful story which will leave the reader wanting to know more."

Dr Julie Coulson, Medical Practioner,
Tusmore, South Australia

"As an author, I know there are many ways to get a message across. On a topic as sensitive as Alzheimer's the message has to be clear, engaging, and give the reader the tools they are seeking. Carolyn has lived her message, and relays it an a style sure to engage you and provide great value. Carolyn's story is a sensitive portrayal of her journey, with all the humour and tribulations of life, and where needed, the candidness to give you a clear message."

Chris Christoff - International author of "Goal Setting for
People Who Can't Set Goals", Project Manager, Property
Investor, IT Professional

"Carolyn's book is truly inspirational and her ability to push through tough times leaves the reader with lots of valuable life lessons on how to overcome adversity, still raise a family and hold down a high level career whilst caring for a loved one. This book has a message in it for everyone."

Darren Stephens, No. 1 Bestselling Author,
'Millionaires & Billionaires Secrets Revealed'

"From great loss can come great learning. "Navigating Alzheimer's" can teach you not just how to survive dementia caring, but how to come out the other end a more resilient and resourceful person."

Sharon Jurd, International Author and Speaker
Australian Franchise Woman of the Year 2014
Qld/NT Franchise Woman of the Year 2014

NAVIGATING
ALZHEIMER'S

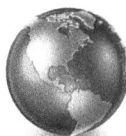

GLOBAL
PUBLISHING
G R O U P

Global Publishing Group
Australia • New Zealand • Singapore • America • London

NAVIGATING ALZHEIMER'S

SURVIVAL SECRETS OF A LONG TERM CARER

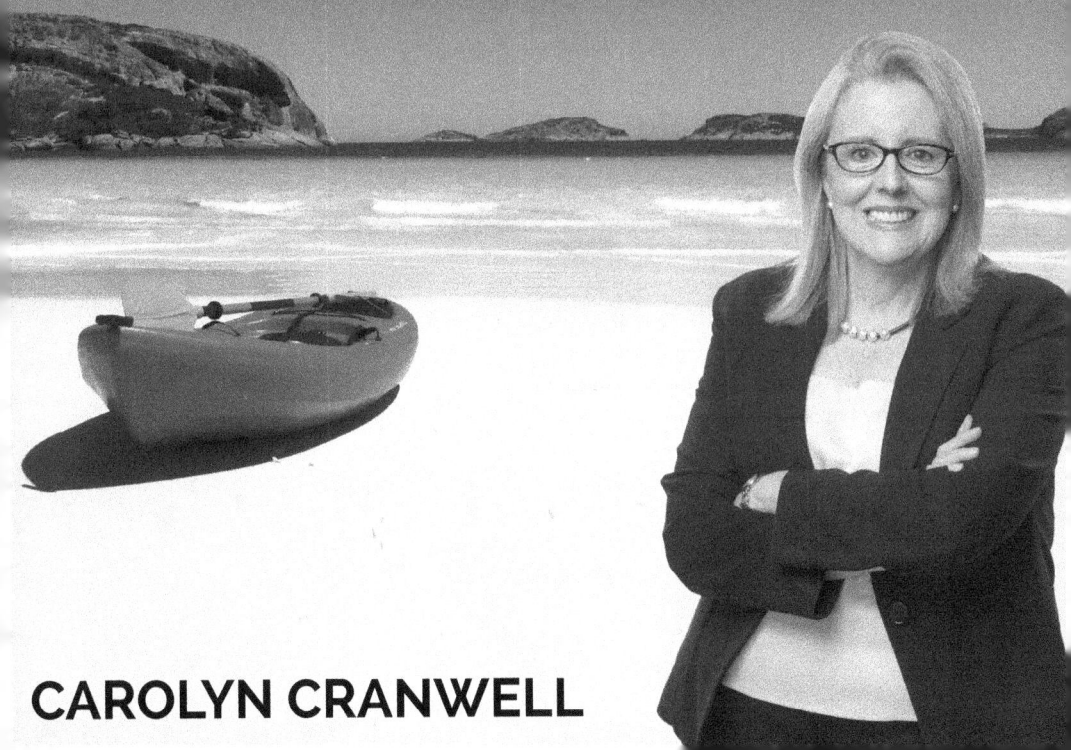

CAROLYN CRANWELL

First Edition 2016

National Library of Australia
Cataloguing-in-Publication entry:

Creator: Cranwell, Carolyn, author.

Navigating Alzheimer's : Survival Secrets Of A Long Term Carer / Carolyn Cranwell.

1st ed.

ISBN: 9781925288254 (paperback)

Alzheimer's disease – Australia.
Alzheimer's disease – Patients--Care – Australia.

Dewey Number: 616.831

Published by Global Publishing Group
PO Box 517 Mt Evelyn, Victoria 3796 Australia
Email info@GlobalPublishingGroup.com.au

Printed in China

For further information about orders:
Phone: +61 3 9739 4686 or Fax +61 3 8648 6871

I dedicate this book to my beloved husband Richard, to our children Ainslie and Jack and to those who stayed close when times got tough.

ACKNOWLEDGEMENTS

This book has been a true labour of love. The inspiration has come from my husband Richard and our children, Ainslie and Jack, whose lives have enriched my life incredibly, giving it true purpose and meaning. I thank you from the bottom of my heart.

I would also like to acknowledge and thank our extended family and friends who supported Richard and accepted him just as he was on any given day no matter what the circumstances.

Alzheimer's is one of the most challenging diseases one can encounter but we did not come through this experience alone. I would like to acknowledge and thank Dr Jane Hecker and Dr Julie Coulson. It was a great comfort and support knowing we were in the hands of such dedicated and supportive medical professionals.

Thank you to all the dedicated carers and volunteers at the dementia day centre and residential facility Richard attended. You are the unsung heroes of this story and deserve recognition. Your genuine interest, professionalism, unfailing patience and friendship with Richard played a major role in his health and wellbeing.

As with any major project, there are a number of incredible people who contributed to making this book happen and I am grateful to all of them.

Thank you to Barbara and John who first suggested I share our story with the world. I dwelled on that thought for a few years but once that idea moved from my heart to my head there was no turning back.

Special thanks to Andrew Jefferis for his guidance and commitment to the book's success and to the inspirational Darren and Jackie Stephens, Kelly and everyone at Global Publishing, for making this dream come true.

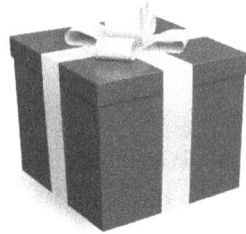

There is so much to learn and understand
about caring for someone with Alzheimer's but there
never seems to be enough hours in the day.

So I have created some reader friendly tips for time poor
carers and other family members and friends to help you
fast track your knowledge and awareness.

- **TOP 10 TIPS:**
  How to communicate with someone with dementia

- **Key Financial and Legal Issues You Should
  Consider**

- **TOP 10 TIPS:**
  How to dementia-proof your home

To Claim Your **FREE BONUS OFFERS** visit...

www.Navigating-Alzheimers.com

CONTENTS

FOREWORD

"Navigating Alzheimer's" provides a fresh, and very personal account of Alzheimer's disease. It is written with truth and honesty but also with a sense of humour, providing hope and inspiration for others. Despite the serious and difficult nature of this disease I found this book very readable and enjoyable. Carolyn has written openly about confronting issues including the veil of secrecy and fear associated with Alzheimer's disease and the sense of isolation that results for families affected by this disease. The insights in this book provide vital understanding, knowledge and direction for all of us who seek to provide support and assistance to family and friends dealing with Alzheimer's disease.

Many of the special issues faced by families affected by younger onset dementia are discussed but most of the issues are equally relevant to older people who develop dementia. "Navigating Alzheimer's" should be essential reading for everyone in the community - for partners and families facing this disease; for those medical, nursing and caring staff working with individuals with Alzheimer's disease and their families; for administrators, funding providers and politicians involved in aged care and health provision; for high school students who need to understand this disease which is increasingly frequent in our community; and for all of us in the community who will come across Alzheimer's disease in our family, our friends and our colleagues.

In many and increasing ways Alzheimer's disease affects us all - this book shows us how to approach this openly and how to provide understanding, practical support and assistance.

Dr Jane Hecker, MBBS (Hons); FRACP; FRCP (UK)
Consultant Physician, Aged Care and Rehabilitation
Special Interest: Memory Disorders

PREFACE

For eighteen years out of our thirty-two year marriage, Richard had Alzheimer's disease. Anyone who has ever tried it will tell you that living with one foot in the past and one foot in the present is an excruciatingly difficult thing to do, but that is the role of a long-term Alzheimer's carer.

For example, try convincing a middle-aged physically healthy independent person that it's time to give up their driving license because they have been diagnosed with a type of dementia known as younger onset Alzheimer's. It's a fast-forward lesson on how to go from hero-to-zero in sixty seconds flat!

At times, the demands of being a primary carer for someone with dementia can be an overwhelming task to the extent that the carer puts their own general health and wellbeing aside and risks becoming a patient themselves. This is particularly so for Alzheimer's carers due to the length and terminal nature of the disease. However, like water dripping on stone, even the strongest constitutions can erode over time.

A carer may have family, employment and financial responsibilities and be operating on a fairly tight timetable. They may be constantly planning ahead to meet daily time frames and future commitments but someone living with Alzheimer's tends to live in the moment and cannot be rushed into action. 'Behavioural forecasts' may be as difficult as the weather to predict, even for experienced carers. Every day is different, bringing its own unique challenges and rewards to the surface. It is just like the John Denver song says, "Some days are diamonds, some days are stone."

A particular feature of long-term caring is that the carers' role and wellbeing are less visible and hidden in the background. Everyone asks after the patient's health but many forget to ask how the carer is managing. The irony of this situation is that in many cases, it is the carer's significant contribution that makes the continuation and daily life of the patient possible and often prevents or delays their entry into a nursing home facility.

Just as a marathon runner requires different skills and attributes from a sprinter, a long-term caring role requires different levels of courage and inner strength from short-term caring. Even the traditional meaning of resilience does not quite fit here because long-term caring is not just a case of step-by-step recovery and gradually "bouncing back" from a one-off event. This is beyond a marathon. For many carers, their responsibilities become a way of life.

Since 2004, my job in State Government has involved providing counter-terrorism policies and advice for public transport systems. Following major international terrorist incidents, government response agencies around the world have enhanced their resilience building strategies and capacity.

Thinking about resiliency at the government and corporate level led me to analyse the culture and behaviour of resilient organisations and consider why some organisations were able to "bounce back" from catastrophic events faster than others. As I deepened my knowledge and understanding of resiliency I observed many similar characteristics amongst resilient organisations and individuals. A strong desire to survive, adapt, grow and move forward was common to all. Parallel to this work, I started thinking about survival skills and resiliency on a personal level and the demanding role of a long-term carer.

A diagnosis of Alzheimer's or any other type of dementia can be incredibly frightening for the person diagnosed but equally so for the person who takes on the primary caring role. They are usually the spouse, partner, children of the couple or sometimes extended family.

But, whose job is it to look after the carer and support them? The answer to this is not quite so clear or easy to define. There are Alzheimer's Associations in Australia and around the world who do wonderful work providing practical information, workshops, support groups and counselling services. Some governments (including the Australian Government) provide assistance with respite services and residential care. Notwithstanding this however, most of the health and support services are directed towards patient care. In writing this book I have directed my thoughts towards the carers' needs and survival.

In reality, survival just comes down to a simple straightforward decision. A conscious act of will might be another way to describe it but whatever you want to call it, it is just a choice......and I chose to survive right from the beginning. I believe that is what kept me strong and what kept us all going. At home we lived in our Alzheimer's bubble but our connection with the outside world, although tenuous at times, is what saved us all from being victims. It also helped my husband enormously. He needed someone to step up and take on his responsibilities.

As life expectancy increases, the health needs created by aging populations is putting additional pressures on families, communities, the public purse, private aged-care providers and the medical and insurance sectors. I believe it's time people started talking openly about Alzheimer's at social gatherings, in the workplace and in the media so that it becomes as commonplace as a discussion about Heart Disease, Cancer or Diabetes. I see this as the only way we will be able to remove the stigma attached to Alzheimer's and other forms of dementia and get the level of support and services that carers need. Until that happens, many carers risk burnout and becoming patients of the health system themselves.

Empower and assist each carer to discover their inner strength and resilience and you strengthen the whole system. Ignore this issue and the risk remains.

OUR STORY

The doctor said, "Richard, you have a progressive degenerative disease of the brain for which there is no cure, no treatment and no operations. There are some drugs which may be helpful in the early stages". In just two sentences... 'Camelot' vanished. The castle walls we had built around our family came tumbling down and all our lives were irrevocably changed forever.

It was February 2003.

I first met Richard in 1979 but it was not until 1981 that we finally met again in the hospitality tent at the Oakbank Easter Race meeting in the Adelaide Hills. Richard bought me a drink which I accepted but when I excused myself to go outside he insisted I stay. He promised to pay me whatever odds the bookies were offering. This continued throughout the afternoon. Every time I went to leave he asked me to stay. I was more than happy to oblige.

The very next day I told my girlfriend Margaret I was absolutely certain that he was the man I was going to marry. After the weekend Richard wanted to send me a gift from Port Lincoln where he lived and I joked saying, "Forget the roses and chocolates, that's so old school, send me a crayfish (lobster)". And to my utter delight and surprise… he did.

My mother knew something was up when out of the blue I showed an interest in cooking. I had formidable competition from the Country Women's Association (CWA) trading stall which appeared on Tasman Terrace, Port Lincoln every Friday morning. Anyone who has ever lived in an Australian country town would know when you are up against the CWA you up against the experts. This called for drastic action. My mother came to the rescue helping me bake two trays of chocolate brownies which I promptly took to the central bus depot marked 'Urgent Delivery' for Mr Richard Cranwell.

After a whirlwind courtship we were engaged four months later in August 1981 and married the following March. We honeymooned in Hawaii.

As newlyweds we spent many happy weekends in and around Port Lincoln on fishing trips, catching delicious King George Whiting, cleaning them on the beach, and making fabulous seafood sandwiches with freshly baked bread and home-made mayonnaise. We moved back to Adelaide in 1983. After selling up in Port Lincoln we returned to Adelaide and bought a semi-renovated house and Richard bought a new business. Our beautiful daughter, Ainslie Elizabeth was born in May 1984 and our son Jack followed in October 1990.

Our lives were simple but complete. During the week we worked and on the weekends we spent time with our children, our parents and friends and renovated our house. Our happiest nights were spent at home after putting the children to sleep. We would order a take-away dinner, open a bottle of beautiful South Australian wine and munch on delicious Haigh's Chocolates while watching a movie. Curtains were usually drawn, lights dimmed and in winter the house was made warm and cosy by a gas heater or a log burning fire. We used to call it 'shutting the rest of the world out'. We were so happy just to be together.

I studied law part-time at university and Richard supported me one hundred percent. When I eventually finished my degree I succeeded in getting a job in government. Two salaries made a difference and put less pressure on Richard and the business.

At that time we had everything in the world - everything that really mattered. We had our love for each other, our health and two beautiful happy children who were doing well at school. Richard was in his early fifties and I was nearly ten years younger. There was no way of seeing the journey that lay ahead.

Sometimes in the morning when Richard left for work he would return to collect things he had forgotten like the business keys, bank books or his lunch. It happened so often that I would wait for the sound of the car braking, the sound of his footsteps in the driveway.

This started to happen more and more frequently so I typed up 'Richard's Check List' and attached it to the inside of our front door. We put all of this down to tiredness and stress from the business. Our Manager, Sherree, advised me that he was struggling a bit at work, being forgetful and having difficulty remembering procedures. Even making relatively simple decisions took longer than usual.

"You two need to go on a holiday. Richard needs a rest from all this", she said.

It was time for us to listen and do more with our lives than just work. In mid-1997 we went on a holiday to Far North Queensland and a year later we attended a business conference in Canada and then spent two weeks travelling through the United States. Both trips were meant to provide a rest from work and stress. However on our return Richard's memory difficulties continued. He didn't seem any better at all. We were aware he was still struggling but he laughed it off and constantly assured me there was nothing to worry about.

It was several years and many forgetful adventures later that I was finally able to convince him he needed to go to the doctor.

In early 2003, after many medical tests we received the diagnosis of younger-onset Alzheimer's disease. I was so naive about this condition at the time that on the drive home from the doctor's office

I assured Richard that this was an older person's disease and that because he was in his early fifties he had years to go before the symptoms manifested themselves. Richard just sat there in silence staring straight ahead. He looked totally confused and shell-shocked.

We arrived home about lunchtime but neither of us could face going back to work. We were renovating our current house for sale while our new home was being built. Our minds were in over-drive after getting the news so we took turns in stripping the wallpaper off the family room walls with a steaming gun. The next day we both returned to work and went on with our lives as if nothing had happened.

Although as shocking as the diagnosis had been it had brought some momentary sense of relief in that the problem had been identified. We weren't just imagining things. We were both determined to fight the disease but were absolutely clueless about what we were up against. That night I came up with a great plan. I would go to the book store the next day on my lunch break and find a book on dementia. We would sit down after dinner and when the children had gone to bed and share a relaxing glass of wine. Then we would go through the text together and get this situation sorted.

However, I had no idea of the surprise that was waiting for me in the book store. I was absolutely aghast when I skimmed the first book I picked up on Alzheimer's. It was a true story about a wife who came home from shopping and found her husband busy painting the walls of their beautiful home with his faeces. This was not the helpful information I was looking for and the next book was even more confronting. Neither was uplifting, encouraging or helpful. I fled the bookstore empty-handed and in a state of sheer panic.

Chapter 1

LOOKING FOR COURAGE

First steps to survival

> "Being deeply loved by someone gives you strength, while loving someone deeply gives you courage."
>
> *Lao Tzu*

Have you ever played that children's birthday party game where there are more children than available chairs? Everyone has to walk around the outer border of the room in a circle. The chairs are positioned in the centre of the room. Music is played and when the music stops the person who doesn't manage to scramble onto a chair and sit down is the one eliminated from the game. That child has to sit out for the rest of the game. This process is repeated until there is only one person left who still has a chair and they are pronounced the winner and given a prize.

Well, that is exactly how we felt after receiving Richard's diagnosis of younger-onset Alzheimer's. We felt as if the music of our life had stopped and we had been left without a chair. There was no soft landing in sight for us. We were chairless and, unlike the party game, there was no waiting until the next round. We could not recoup our losses when 'pass-the-parcel' or 'pin-the-tail-on-the-donkey' came around. We had to continue our lives as best we could. This was our new reality.

Approximately every twelve to eighteen months we visited Richard's doctor and Richard's Mini Mental State Exam (MMSE) test results for memory and cognitive skills continued to plummet.

His first score was 23/30, then progressively, 19/30, followed by 16/30, and eventually 7/30. The questions were wide ranging: "spell the word 'world' backwards... count down from 100 in sevens i.e. 100, 97, 90." Another part of the test involved Richard having to draw the hands on a clock face e.g. 2:10pm. The first few visits he managed to complete the clock. This was reassuring. I thought, "Great. He can still tell the time," but this skill had evaporated by the time our next visit came around. Instead of filling in the time, Richard drew a series of concentric circles inside the clock face. On a subsequent visit he picked up the pen but then put it down and ignored it. To my astonishment he started using his index finger like a pen. He proceeded to attempt writing the clock task with his finger moving slowly across the page. It was heartbreaking to watch.

At first the diagnosis had come as something of a relief. Now we had a road map for the future but the reality took a lot longer to sink in. My brief panic in a bookstore, when I fled in shock after scanning some of the medical books about Alzheimer's, was nothing compared to the sense of overwhelming fear I experienced when I realised the nature of what lay ahead. It was more than just 'losing the chairs we were sitting on,' it was as if the ground beneath us had disappeared. I could see the fear and uncertainty in Richard's and the children's eyes and the emotional pain I felt when I witnessed this was far worse for me than any physical pain I had ever previously endured.

The more I thought about the challenges that lay ahead for Richard and the family I couldn't help but wonder where I would find the courage, strength and energy to get us safely through this crisis.

I believe the starting point was realising that we were facing an uncertain future which, if not handled carefully, had the power to tear us apart. I couldn't stand by and let that happen - not on my watch. There was no question about commitment. I resolved to do everything in my power to keep us together as a family and keep Richard at home for as long as possible. I knew he would do the same for me without having to think twice. I knew I might one day have to admit Richard to a nursing home. This prospect chilled me to the bone but I tried not to dwell on it and to focus on the present situation - one crisis at a time.

After the diagnosis, how we would cope was my primary concern. I never really bothered about 'why' this had happened to us. There was simply no point. It would not have achieved anything and only provided more stress. There was no family history of dementia and Richard was a non-smoker, moderate drinker, he had a good weight and led a healthy lifestyle. There was little ambiguity in the diagnosis either. The doctor had made the situation crystal clear. We could not negotiate our way around this. The results were in and Richard exhibited every clinical factor indicating Alzheimer's. I had taken Richard to all of his medical appointments and been with him for every test, examination and brain scan and the possibility of mistaken diagnosis seemed unlikely.

As frightening and confronting as I found watching Richard undergo the CT scan, I am glad I witnessed it and saw the results. It really helped me by seeing the physical signs of deterioration. Richard's brain looked like a page from a street directory, except where there should have been a clear flow of traffic from one 'road' to another, his arteries appeared blocked and damaged. They reminded me of streets bearing signs saying, 'Detour Next 2 Kilometres, Bridge Out of Service,' or 'Do Not Take Freeway Due to Fog' or 'Road-works Ahead Take Alternative Route.' A sticky plaque-like 'fog' had settled on parts of Richard's brain and it was causing havoc with his communication, thinking and memory systems. Now I understood why Richard was having trouble taking information in and communicating his thoughts outwardly. His brain was having a traffic jam!

Seeing those scans made it crystal clear that it was absolutely futile wasting any time agonising over why this had happened to Richard and our family. After approximately five years of escalating uncertainty the evidence was finally there. We just had to accept it and move on. That's not to say there weren't plenty of tears at times. We all had our moments and I spent many nights soaking my pillow after Richard and the children were fast asleep. My puffy eyes the next morning were passed off as hay fever or allergy. This seemed to satisfy everyone and so we continued with our daily routines.

When I came home in the evening there were meals to prepare and all the usual distractions of a normal active family to occupy my time. At night, when the house was quiet and before I fell asleep was really the only time I had to myself to think without interruptions. It was during those rare moments of silence that I thought about how I was going to solve this unsolvable situation. The harder I tried to think of practical solutions the more I came up blank.

However, one thought that did keep coming back to me was that I was going to need a lot of courage.

"Great," I thought. "I'll just run down to the supermarket and pick up a few kilos of courage. That will come in handy when Richard asks me the same question five times in a row, when the car keys go missing again or when the children look at me to see why their Dad is acting so out of character."

What worried me most and kept me awake at night in the early post-diagnosis days was where or how I would find the inner strength to sustain us year after year. Could it even be for a decade or more? We were facing a marathon, not a sprint and as every long distance runner will tell you - that takes an entirely different mindset.

I was so scared for all of us that in my mind, courage became a tangible thing. I just had to get some. I knew if I could find it we could face anything. I became obsessed with my search for the source of courage.

My first lesson about courage, although I didn't realise it at the time, came from my parents. I was six years old when I tripped while playing at a neighbour's house and severely dislocated my left hip. At the outset, the doctors had advised my parents that I would never be able to walk again without the aid of crutches and a special built up boot and that they should place me in a home for crippled children. My mother refused to take their advice and nursed me at home.

After months spent in a plaster cast, followed by intensive physiotherapy at home, the doctors pronounced that I was completely healed and that with practice I would be able to walk normally again. My parents were elated. I was also excited but I couldn't understand what all the big fuss was about. In my childish mind it was never a question of if I would walk again, it was only a matter of time. We were just waiting for the 'green light' or so I thought. After all, I was ready! Plaster cast off, physio done and everyone around me was calm, supportive and loving. Going back to school and catching up with my friends was foremost in my mind and I just assumed everything would return to normal.

Looking back now, I realise that I held that blind faith because I simply had no reason for doubt. I was totally unaware of the doctor's prognosis and I never saw any fear in my parents' faces. I am not sure if it was the strength of my mother's religious beliefs, my parents' binding love for each other, their burning desire to protect me or a combination of all three but something gave them that internal fortitude. The memory of the way in which they coped with my accident was not lost on me many years later when I was facing my own 'Mount Everest' of fear.

There are plenty of examples of people who have done brave things in the world and if I could just discover what their secret was then I could use it to help my family survive.

As a teenager, I was interested in reading about people who had conquered their own fears. I remember reading about Thor Heyerdahl, the Norwegian adventurer and the true story of his Kon-Tiki Expedition – his epic journey sailing 8,000 kilometres across the Pacific Ocean, from South America to the Tuamotu Islands, French Polynesia, in a hand built raft made of reeds. How does someone do that, I wondered? How do they literally let go of the shore?

Hyerdahl had a clear objective in mind when he started out on his epic journey and I realised I needed one too. You might think that was obvious but when you are as shell shocked by the diagnosis as we were, it was difficult to hang any label on a situation that didn't seem to have any boundaries or timelines. I wanted to navigate my family safely through Alzheimer's. It was as simple and as complex as that. There were only two words that sprang to mind: courage and survival.

We all needed to survive in our separate ways but I felt responsible for all of us. The way Richard looked at me, he didn't have to say any words. His thoughts were written in his eyes. His look was his cry for help and I could tell he was voluntarily handing over the reins. He was struggling to come to terms with his changing reality and he needed space to do that without having to worry about everyday domestic responsibilities and duties or how his family was coping with the changing of the guard.

Whenever I thought about survival during those private moments at night, a particular picture of my family often appeared in my mind like a recurring dream. I'm not sure if it was Thor Heyerdahl's influence or not but we were all sitting in a small dinghy and we were heading across open water towards a beach where we would land. There was nothing familiar or remarkable about where we were going but I just knew I was intent on getting us there. I sat in the stern of the boat steering, while Richard sat on the plank in the middle and the children sat together in the bow. No one ever said anything. We rode across the water in stony silence, all of us lost in our own thoughts, not looking at each other, just staring straight ahead.

There was only one thought in my mind the whole time we were in the boat and it kept playing over and over again like a sound loop:

"I have to get us safely to the shore."
"I have to get us safely to the shore."
"I have to get us safely to the shore."

In daylight I translated this to mean I had to get Richard, Jack and Ainslie where they all needed to be. For Richard this was to be in a more accepting peaceful frame of mind and eventually, when I could no longer look after him at home, into residential care and for Jack and Ainslie it was through school, university and onwards into fulfilling lives. This picture was so vivid in my mind that I was able to recall it whenever I felt the need and it stayed with me throughout our entire Alzheimer's journey. I still see it now as clearly as the first day it appeared. The 'sea journey' dream helped me clarify what I had to do but I still didn't feel I had the courage and strength to get us 'safely to the shore.' Our lives had dramatically changed to alter our expectations of life as we knew it.

Anyone who had ever met Richard would wholeheartedly agree that he was one of the most unselfish people that you could ever hope to meet so I knew with absolute certainty that he would have wanted Ainslie and Jack to lead the lives they would have led if he had not got Alzheimer's. We might have tip-toed around the subject but we never really discussed that specific point at any length because it was so strongly implied by his personality, character and values.

Richard was aware of his future but talking about it in detail was so confronting and frightening for him that we touched the surface lightly. I could see that to delve further into an uncertain future would have been even more destabilising in circumstances that were already fragile at best. Our everyday lives had become caught in a time warp of fast forward in the real world and slow motion in Richard's world. At times we engaged in that most difficult of all balancing acts - walking a tightrope between the two. We continued to go through the everyday motion of our lives and I tried hard to ignore the constantly nagging voice inside me that questioned whether I was up to the task or not.

I had embarked on a long-term goal once before when I was studying for my law degree part time over a number of years so I wasn't a total stranger to long-term commitment. Studying law was something I had undertaken voluntarily for a set period of time (eight years) and there was a positive reward at the end for all the years of hard work. Richard's situation was the complete opposite. There was nothing voluntary about it and there was no finite timeframe for Alzheimer's. A typical prognosis for someone with younger-onset Alzheimer's is six to eight years but there have been cases where people have lived nearly twenty years after diagnosis. We had no way of knowing whether we were facing a 'sprint' or a 'marathon,' although neither was going to be easy.

I started thinking back to that time when I had struggled with self-belief as a student. There had been times towards the end of my degree when I wondered if I was ever going to make it. Ainslie had just started school and Jack was a non-sleeping baby until he was ten months old. There were so many competing priorities from children through to grandparents. Could I stay focused? Did I have what it took to finish what I had started? How much did I want to achieve this goal? Well, I was so far in that quitting was just not an option but I knew I was tiring and badly in need of a confidence boost.

My nights were mostly sleepless anyway so I had plenty of time to reflect.

I remembered when I was studying American History I came across a delightful book written by the renowned British journalist and radio broadcaster, Alistair Cooke. Being a journalist and amateur historian, Cooke indulged his passion for both art forms in print and radio. He shared his love of American history and gift with words with his hungry fans in 1973, when he published "Alistair Cooke's America." I loved Cooke's signature trademark of laconic, understated style and thrifty economical use of words which is as obvious throughout the three hundred and ninety-five pages, as greasy fingerprints over a crime scene.

It was such a pleasant change from law. The more I read the more I could feel Cooke reeling me in. His unique take on life made the past come alive. No chapter was more compelling for me than his account of Abraham Lincoln's ascension to President. Here Cooke interweaves the history of the American Civil War with his extraordinary insight into the personality and character of a man regarded as one of America's greatest Presidents.

It is no secret that Lincoln was not always seen as a hero. In fact, until he reached his middle years he was widely regarded as more of a failure than a success. History tells us that when he finally did succeed he exceeded everyone's expectations, including his own. This aspect of Lincoln's life fascinated me. How could someone who had failed in business, faced defeat regularly and consistently in politics and suffered a nervous breakdown turn out to be such a runaway success? How was this possible? Where did he find the courage to repeatedly risk ridicule and failure?

Cooke was also intrigued by Lincoln's litany of struggles and eventual metamorphic journey towards success when he wrote:

"By some brain chemistry that has never been explained, Lincoln transformed in middle life his whole style of speaking and writing.

His early speeches are frontier-lawyer baroque, stuffed with the fustian of his time. We know that he steeped himself in the subtleties of Shakespeare, the cadences of the Bible, and the hard humanity of Robert Burns. And somehow, and conspicuously during the war, he became what he always must have been: a shrewd, honourable frontiersman of very great gifts."

These words haunted me and I kept reading this paragraph over and over again. Something about Lincoln's transformation rattled me. I couldn't work out what was bothering me but at the same time I just couldn't let it go. It became a mild form of obsession, an itch that I couldn't scratch.

Eventually one phrase stood out. I felt the words almost leap off the page:

"..... he became what he always must have been......"

The words kept going around and around in my head......."he became what he always must have been.....he became what he always must have been."

This dragged on for days. It became my new mantra.

But what did it really mean? I washed dishes thinking about this. I bought groceries, I did housework, I went to university, I studied law and I cooked meals, distracted by these thoughts. How could anyone be such a consistent failure and then turn into such a widely acclaimed success?

As a circuit breaker I shifted my fixation away from Cooke's 'riddle' and focused on Lincoln's impressive catalogue of failures. This proved to be safer ground. There were enough bona fide failures there to make most of us feel good about ourselves for many years to come! In fact, I was so heartened by Lincoln's dubious track record that I began to relax a little and see things more clearly.

It wasn't until I started seeing each of his failures as stepping stones to success that I made any headway with the puzzle. I could see Lincoln's persistence definitely played a part. Once I headed down that track I saw the answer had been right in front of me, hiding in plain sight. Lincoln had what I call the 'raw ingredients' to become President right from the beginning and they were present, although not evident, all through his epic failures. They just got refined and moulded along the way. His struggles were the source of his strength. Overcoming them became a way of life.

A strong work ethic, the ability to focus and a dogged determination to succeed had landed him fair and square in the winner's circle. In the end....."he became what he always must have been, a shrewd, honourable frontiersman of very great gifts." Clearly, Lincoln's eventual success came from his inner strength. No matter what the circumstances, he became his own source of courage, strength and power, his own living unbreakable chain of momentum.

That was it. The elusive answer to Cooke's riddle was now clear to me. If it was true for Lincoln, could it not be true for all of us? If I applied Lincoln's example to my own life, could I simply fail my way to success? All along I had been looking for the answer but always searching outwardly for the source of courage, never dreaming of looking inwardly. Cooke and Lincoln had taught me that I already had everything I needed. Now, I just had to find a way to bring this courage to the surface.

What a relief. Well, a relief of course until little niggling doubts began to raise their heads. Will I have the courage when I need it? How much will I need? Could I ever be like Lincoln and come back time after time when faced with significant loss, disappointment or outright defeat?

I was still mulling over all this when I remembered a story from my childhood which suddenly calmed me and gave me hope. When I was five years old I learned that the mother of one of my school friends was having a baby. My friend was very underwhelmed by the news of the impending new arrival, as was I. Life as we knew it was under threat. My friend's security in the family pecking order was about to be swept away by some silly stork - a bird that can't even fly!

Concerned that this stork might be in the neighbourhood and could also make an unwelcome visit to my house, I confronted my mother as soon as I got home.

"What if a mother had another baby? What would happen to the other children? Who would look after and love them?"

My mother took a while to think about this and then answered, "Oh that's easy. If a new baby comes along, the mother just makes some more love for the new baby. There is still plenty of love to go around for all the children. A mother just keeps making more love for each new baby that comes along."

I was so happy with this answer, I just said, "Thanks Mum" and without another thought or concern I ran outside to play with my neighbours.

I couldn't wait to get to school the next day to break the news to my nervous friend that everything was going to be alright. Situation 'Unwelcome Stork' had been sorted.

So I started wondering if courage and inner strength are like love. If you need some more courage, perhaps you just make some more. If we accept that the raw source of courage comes from within us, perhaps all we need to do is dig deeper when pushed. I found this idea immensely comforting. If it was anything like my mother's love then the source of my new courage would be endless.

I can do this! I can get my family 'safely to the shore.'

TAKE-AWAYS

CHAPTER 1

- The diagnosis comes as a shock but it's rarely a surprise

- Everyone can be distracted and forget. When it falls into patterns you need to investigate

- Look for survival signs from your past - your history - the past to teach us the future - the past points to the future

- We all have the raw ingredients for courage

- Our strength increases as we overcome our struggles

- Failure is but a stepping stone to success

- Courage comes from within

Chapter 2

PUTTING ON A BRAVE FACE

Living with the 'Crisis-du-Jour'

> "Nothing in this world can take the place of persistence. Talent will not, nothing is more common than unsuccessful men with talent. Genius will not, unrewarded genius is almost a proverb. Education will not, the world is full of educated derelicts. Persistence and determination alone are omnipotent."
>
> *Calvin Coolidge*

As Richard's disease progressed we seemed to lurch from one crisis to the next, ranging from frustrating domestic events to a life threatening heart attack, violent seizures and falls in the later stages. Living in crisis mode became the new normal. I got so used to dealing with crisis on a daily basis that I named these phenomena the '*Crisis-du-Jour.*'

For all of us, the home front went from being a place of refuge to unfamiliar territory. For me it felt like Alzheimer's had kidnapped my husband and held the rest of the family to ransom. Every day was unpredictable and would relentlessly serve up a menu of totally random events. We could rarely just get up and get ready for work or school without some unfortunate incident taking place.

Richard began to need help with dressing and grooming. Small things we take for granted like doing up buttons and tying shoelaces started to present considerable challenges. He often tried to accomplish these tasks but it was too difficult for him to use a toothbrush, shaving stick or a hairbrush. I tried to stay focussed at work but during the day I frequently started wondering what I would face when I walked through the front door that night.

Compulsive anticipation often becomes part of the primary carer's mindset.

When Richard was still living at home it was suggested to me one day that I keep a diary to record all the stories and incidents that happened to us during that time in case I wanted to refer to them later. "I don't have to" I replied, "this is my whole life, I won't forget it. I have lived this story 24/7. Name any room or space in the house or garden and I can tell you a story about Richard's struggle with Alzheimer's."

Mornings were stressful but evenings weren't any better.

One particular night will stand out in our memory forever. I had no sooner walked across the front door mat when I could sense the tension in the air. The feeling was radiating off the walls. I could hear raised voices as I walked down our long hallway to a scene of chaos in the kitchen. A pan on the stove was bubbling away furiously. Richard was wandering around in circles looking confused and highly agitated while two very distraught young faces were staring at their father in disbelief.

As I approached I could see that chicken schnitzels were happily cooking in the pan but a sea of sizzling foam had engulfed them and was about to boil over. An innocent bottle of golden liquid was sitting quietly nearby on the kitchen bench as if unaware that it was the cause of such commotion. I knew immediately what had happened. It was heart breaking. Richard was trying so hard to help by having dinner ready for us. This was typical of his loving and thoughtful nature. It was even more tragic because it was plain to see that he was desperately trying to show us he could still cope with normal everyday tasks. His best intentions had backfired when he had mistaken the contents of the bottle. What appeared to him to be a bottle of cooking oil was in fact a bottle of yellow dishwashing detergent left out unintentionally on the bench near the hotplates. We had to be more vigilant now.

Chicken schnitzels were a family dinnertime favourite and guaranteed to bring smiles all round - but not that evening. "At least we have a very clean frying pan," I quipped, but no one had much of an appetite left for food or laughter.

Another difficulty arose, this time with the toaster. Richard had buttered toast but then forgot he had buttered it and had put it back into the toaster to cook again. I was pleased and proud that he was still trying to be independent but when the smoke from the burnt butter started to fill the kitchen and slowly spread through the house I got really worried. I could easily air the house but the risk of fire was a far greater concern. After that incident we had to be so careful all the time. I put the toaster away in a cupboard out of sight and only brought it out at breakfast.

The control panel on the new dishwasher was digital. Oh my… so many buttons and flashing lights. It was all very confusing. Richard was so keen to help me with the dishes that in the end, out of sheer frustration, he used to push all the buttons all at once which apparently left the computer in the control panel confused too and the brand new machine 'spat the dummy' and refused to wash any dishes.

A week later, an expensive visit from the repair man sorted the issue out but it left Richard gun-shy of the dishwasher and me racking my brain for non-electrical chores that he could complete successfully and from which he could derive some satisfaction and pleasure.

The refrigerator broke down on one New Year's Day in the middle of a heatwave. As I walked down our hallway towards our kitchen I noticed that the hall rug had been moved. I called out, "Why did you shift the rug?" As soon as I turned the corner into the kitchen I knew the answer. I was standing in icy cold water. Our refrigerator had 'died' overnight and everything was melting. Richard's reply was, "I shifted the rug because the floor was wet." He had prepared his bowl of cereal and was now happily munching it nearby. It had not occurred to him to investigate the cause or source of the puddle.

At that point I realised he was 'on the last step of the ladder' as far as logic was concerned. He could do no more than recognise that the floor was wet. He was incapable of thinking the rest of the situation through to a resolution. We had to live out of an ice box for weeks - there were no refrigerators available for hire in the whole of the city. Spare parts took another three weeks and they arrived just as the cool change kicked in.

One member of the family I haven't mentioned was Harry our dog. Harry and Richard were great mates. It seemed that walking Harry around the block was an enjoyable and helpful task for Richard to do. Not to forget that I could always rely on Harry to bring his master safely home. He loved these walks with Richard and would wait by his lead whenever he spotted it. They were both pleased to settle down on the sofa on their return, happy to just hang out together. These adventures with Harry around our neighbourhood gave Richard a little dose of unsupervised freedom and a sense of independence which was a real boost to his ego and spirits.

Their sphere also extended to the garden. Richard was born in the country so he loved being outside and he was very happy to spend many hours outside watering with Harry. Although this arrangement could not continue forever, it was a wonderful time for both of them while it lasted.

I came home one evening to find Harry and Richard in front of the television. It was a lovely peaceful sight. Harry was laid out at Richard's feet and snoring contentedly with (unbeknownst to me) a very full stomach. Richard had opened the fridge and obviously discovered the family's lamb and vegetable casserole I had made the night before. He had given the entire meal to a grateful Harry for his dinner. Both were blissfully unaware that a sudden menu change for the family was about to happen but that was ok. Baked beans on toast to the rescue once again!

So inadvertently, Harry felt the impact of Richard's illness. Being a Labrador, Harry was certainly not complaining about the extra care and meals he was receiving. Clearly eating in moderation was not remotely on his radar; no canine weight-watching for him. Eventually, a visit to the vet and a stringent diet and exercise plan were the result of Harry's frequent over-indulgence, although who can actually blame him?

Incidents like this happened so frequently that I stopped cooking meals in advance and started cooking when I got home from work. This was a less than ideal arrangement but too many family meals had disappeared down the vast food disposal system otherwise known as Harry.

About the time Harry became the beneficiary of our family dinners another extraordinary event occurred. Our house fell victim to the notorious 'Ice-Cream Bandit.' A mysterious and unpopular villain raiding our refrigerator and robbing us of our night time treat. Previously, a two-litre tub of French vanilla bought on Saturday would normally last to the following weekend but once the bandit arrived on the scene, our precious supplies could run out at any time. This caused considerable angst amongst all family members. However, despite a security alert and interrogation session conducted by me, no guilty party was forth-coming. Everyone was immediately running for cover and of course vehemently denying culpability. To this day, I'm still unsure of the culprit but it just may have been a tall human with a canine accomplice.

I had mistakenly thought our new house would be easy for Richard but instead, it proved quite the opposite and presented many difficulties. We noticed that he was looking for the kettle and toaster in the new kitchen as if he was in the old, now demolished, house and they were now in the left-hand corner, not the right.

Frequently, Richard would stand by the stove at night when we all got home. He was eager to help but as it became more and more difficult I had to deflect his enthusiasm. One night I hit upon a great idea. "How about you read the paper at the table and see what's in the news." He always enjoyed the paper and so he would sit and just turn over the pages only looking at the photographs and pictures.

There were inevitably many more domestic adventures in other parts of the house however, the kitchen and family room stands out because it was the focus of activity every morning and evening and the one place where the whole family gathered. It is a place where you are acutely aware of someone's ability to function and to the state of their wellbeing. For us, Richard's decline (a suspicion well before the diagnosis and a confirmation from day one) was made most apparent in and around the kitchen.

We often found that if we didn't overreact we could be more tolerant and just get on with the day. If you found a glass of left-over wine covered in plastic clingwrap in the microwave or the ice cream melting in the pantry you just smiled to yourself and made a mental note that Richard had started to lose his understanding of the purpose of cupboards and fridges. When I inevitably got to the stage of employing carers in our home each weekday I had to teach them to just 'smile and get on with it' as we had learnt.

Support in helping me survive during this time came from an unexpected source. I was aware I needed to keep up my appearance and *'put on a brave face'*

I could often see the fear in everyone's eyes, including Richard's. We did not talk about it much because we were constantly in survival mode but I knew just how much they were depending on me to hold the family together. I thought that if I went 'down' we would all go down and I am not sure how long it would have taken us to bounce back. One thing I was sure about was that if I looked ok it would give the family confidence and confidence was something we were all struggling to maintain. If I had dark rings from lack of sleep and black racoon eyes from tear smudged mascara it would be a definite giveaway that I wasn't coping too well and Richard would pick up on this. He would know something was wrong but he would not know what exactly or how to fix it. So every morning I applied my make-up like I was painting on a protective mask.

My two favourite products were *Maybelline Waterproof Mascara* and *Maybelline Erase* – for covering dark circles under the eyes and camouflaging other skin flaws. They worked a treat! I still use them today.

Every morning when the family's day had been started in the kitchen I would retreat back to the bathroom and put on my 'mask' for the day and thus fortified, I would sally forth to face whatever 'Crisis du Jour' the day would throw at me.

TAKE-AWAYS

CHAPTER 2

- Early signs become important later

- Adjust your living space and put away some kitchen appliances if necessary

- Rethink all of your routines around the home

- Looking good makes you feel good and gives other family members confidence in you

Chapter 3

THE LITTLE BLUE BOOK AND THE CHEESE PIZZA

Travelling overseas

> "Only those who risk going too far can possibly find out
> how far they can go."
>
> *T.S. Eliot*

In 2002, about a year before Richard's diagnosis of Alzheimer's, we went on an amazing overseas holiday with some friends. Our plan was to spend a few days in London before heading off to the stunning west coast of Ireland and then on to the beautiful UNESCO World Heritage township of Sintra, in Portugal.

Richard had lived in London in his early twenties but I had never been there before so I was very excited. He had promised to show me around and be my personal tour guide. We were the advance scouts for our group, being the first to arrive in London. We checked into our hotel in Kensington and then headed straight out to explore the streets. We hadn't walked very far at all when a 'hop-on-hop-off' bus pulled up right in front of us. It was too tempting to refuse as we were jetlagged and all of our energy was adrenalin driven.

There was so much to see and take in! We sat upstairs for the best view. I had looked forward to this trip for ages and I didn't want to miss a moment. We completed the first full loop, whizzing past Buckingham Palace, the London Eye, Big Ben and the Tower Bridge but when we arrived back at the change-over stop for the alternative line, Richard suggested we stay on the same bus and go around again. "Okay," I thought, "a good way for us to get orientated." The weather had turned a little cool and the bus was warm and cosy so round we went again. I was puzzled by Richard's reticence but just put it down to tiredness from the long haul flight.

We switched route lines and the next bus we got on headed down Regent Street. Richard became very excited when he recognised the Café Royal. He had worked there for about eighteen months back in the early seventies. His reaction was so animated that it was as if he was greeting the Café Royal like a long lost friend, which indeed he was......

The Café Royal was the only landmark that had really resonated with Richard that afternoon, despite having seen many famous sights, most of which he would have seen before. And of course he wanted to go around again so he could see the Café Royal one more time.

I agreed, hoping that would settle him down a little but he reacted with the same excitement when we hit Regent Street. This behaviour was starting to scare me and by then I was desperate to get us off the bus.

The bus ticket included a cruise down the Thames but this was rejected outright. A ride on the London Eye was also not a winner. Apart from my disappointment, when I asked Richard if he would like to do either of those activities tomorrow, his response was even more alarming. He said he needed more time. "How much more time?" I asked. "Oh about a week…..If we were here for a week… …I could do it...... but I need more time." We only had a day and a half in London so that was not possible.

This wasn't the Richard I knew. I couldn't understand why he was acting so out of character. Perhaps the strain of leaving the business and the flight was more stressful than I realised or was it just the "push-pull" effect of such a large city? "Better head back to the hotel," I thought. An early dinner and a good night's sleep would sort things out, I hoped.

We were only back a short while when our friends arrived. With the familiar faces and the quiet comfort of the hotel surroundings, Richard was back to his normal self again. Phew! I was relieved because I was beginning to think earlier that afternoon that I was travelling with a complete stranger.

I made an executive decision the next morning to have a quiet day and Richard was more than happy with this idea. A casual walk around Kensington proceeded by a long leisurely lunch was just the right pace. I am sure there were snails who meandered faster than us that day but it was a stress-free time and a good circuit breaker before our flight out the next morning to rejoin our group in Ireland.

The next morning we took the Piccadilly line to Heathrow early enough to check-in our luggage and then settle down to a relaxing coffee and some serious people watching.

As we pulled out of the Gloucester Road tube station I couldn't help but reflect on the journey so far. Nothing had turned out quite how I had anticipated. Many hours spent together around the kitchen table planning our brief but exciting visit to London had produced nothing but a series of blurred images of the exterior facades of some of London's highlights. Our usual "hit-the-ground-running holiday strategy" style had not got out of the starting blocks. The hop-on-hop-off repetitive loop scheme didn't really count as 'exploring' in my view but Richard seemed totally oblivious to any shortcomings. Having left London behind, we were both looking forward tremendously to our week in Ireland and the company of our friends and as Richard's behaviour was starting to make me nervous, I was looking forward to the comfort of their support.

Heathrow was its usual chaotic self, rowdy and smelly and teeming with assorted nationalities and their dialects. I was a little apprehensive. Without consciously realising it, I was already trying to anticipate Richard's needs as I could see he was somewhat stressed.

We managed to check in our luggage and although we had to queue we sailed through security without a mishap. We had plenty of time to spare so we began wandering through the duty free shops and had fun comparing prices and converting them to Australian dollars.

We sniffed exotic French perfumes, tasted delicious Swiss chocolate samples and tried on designer sunglasses to while away the time. Tired of window shopping we found a cosy little coffee shop and I asked Richard to mind the bags while I ordered and paid for the coffees. I didn't want any mishaps before boarding the plane so I made sure I had an unobstructed direct line of sight to Richard and the bags. I waved and he smiled back at me seeming quite relaxed.

The café was busy so the coffees took a little longer than expected but we had nothing else to do so what did it matter? After a delicious cappuccino I did a routine check for our boarding passes and passports just to be sure everything was in order.

But everything was not in order!

There were two boarding passes and only one passport. "Stay calm," I told myself, "stay calm".....don't let Richard see that you are alarmed.....plaster a smile on your face and leave it there until the disobedient passport turns up.....smile confidently but keep checking every pocket and every compartment of handbag and carry-on luggage." A thorough check of all our pockets and luggage compartments turned up nothing. I repeated this process and still drew a blank.

Richard sensed something was up so I explained what had happened. "Don't worry, I'll find it," I said, although not feeling overly confident. The seed of doubt that had begun to sprout in my stomach the moment I discovered the loss, had grown into a giant Moreton Bay fig tree by now. My blood pressure was no doubt rising and my heart was starting to pound so loudly I was surprised other customers hadn't turned around to see what was making so much noise.

My personal version of a 'customs search' had produced no results. The genuine fear in my voice was obvious to me, if not to Richard. It was now approximately a little over one hour before we were due to board our flight. I was struggling to keep myself composed.

As much as I was trying to hold things together my mildly frenzied activity probably gave the game away and it was clear that Richard's anxiety was rising in direct proportion to my own. Nothing for it. I realised we would just have to retrace our steps and go back to every duty free shop we had visited, which we proceeded to do. Only this time, the waft of sweet smelling scents that had previously delighted us was now just an annoyance and in fact, rather nauseating. We rushed from perfumes to confectionery and finally to accessories. There were queues of happy travellers with time on their hands in each shop. That was us about sixty agonising minutes ago. I didn't know how much longer I could keep up the pretence and keep reassuring Richard that everything was going to be alright.

I tried to wait patiently but minutes seemed like hours until finally our turn arrived and I asked the smiling assistant if any passports had been handed in during the last hour. "No, sorry Luv," was the hasty reply before moving on to the next customer. When we had entirely retraced our steps and come to the last of the duty free shops my nerves were quite shattered. Our flight was due to board in under an hour.

I cannot to this day remember which passport was missing, it didn't really matter anyway, but Richard turned to me and said, "Darling, what's the matter? What's wrong?" I could tell by the expression on his face that he had totally forgotten the passport was missing. It was unbelievable. He had some understanding that something was not right but no real appreciation of the tight situation we were in. I could not comprehend his state of mind but I had no time to really consider it anyway.

To compound matters, there were logistical hurdles with no immediate solution. It was 2002 and we didn't have iPhones. There was no way of communicating with our friends waiting in Ireland. They were driving from Connemara on the west coast to pick us up from Shannon Airport, in Galway. Finances were also an issue. We weren't exactly flush with funds and every option I could think of was incredibly expensive. While there was some contingency in our holiday budget, an extended stay in London waiting for a new passport to be issued was not something we had factored into our spending money.

I could not recall ever being in such a difficult situation in my life.

No obvious solution was forthcoming. We just stood in the middle of the concourse and let the steady sea of passengers circumnavigate around us. It turned out standing still and breathing deeply was the best thing we could have done. I looked left to right and left again, like a seven year-old learning to cross the road.

On my left I could see a steady flow of passengers coming through passport control. I wondered...just maybe? I was convinced we had both passports when we had toured the shops and so we must have lost one there but by this time I was so beside myself I was ready to try anything. I waited until there was a slight pause in the line-up and nervously approached one of the customs officers.

Somehow I managed to get the words out, "Excuse me Sir, has anyone handed in a passport?"

The officer just looked at us and seemed to sense our silent panic.

"What colour, lady?" My heart skipped a beat. "Blue," I gulped. It felt as if all the air had been sucked out of my lungs. "Wait here," he said and spun around only to return moments later waving a little blue book bearing the Australian coat of arms on the cover.

My smile muscles and vocal chords were almost frozen. It was all I could do to get out a shaky, "Thank you" while still trying to keep the lid on my emotional pressure-cooker.

It was my Judy Dench, Merrill Streep and Cate Blanchett moment rolled into one. A giant wave of relief welled up inside me and a few tears escaped down my cheek - not quite the Oscar-winning performance I was striving for - but close enough. I quickly wiped the tears away and thanks to my trusty *Maybelline Waterproof Mascara* no unsightly evidence remained. I turned to Richard and flashed a smile which he promptly returned. He was happy that I appeared happy. "Everything is alright now," I said as confidently as I could. Then I took him by the arm and we headed for the departure gate where a steady line-up was forming. We found two seats side-by-side and sat there, not daring to move until the flight was called. Crisis averted, but I was wondering what was happening to my husband.

The custom's officer had said that the passport had been dropped just a few feet from the control desk and had been safe sitting in the office waiting to be reclaimed. It was all coming back to me now, like a slow motion movie in replay. I remember thinking that Richard was struggling with the airport environment so I presented our passports and boarding passes while at the same time I was also juggling my shoulder bag, a small case on wheels, both our jackets, and Richard's small cabin bag. No wonder one of the passports had fallen out of my hands and slipped silently to the floor.

Sitting on the plane to Ireland and mulling over our close escape from disaster, I realised our travel arrangements from here on needed to radically change. Little did I know at the time that it wasn't just our travel arrangements. Nothing would escape unscathed. We were like a pair of amateur mountaineers stranded on a precipice. The rocky outcrop was camouflaging the sheer drop below.

Not surprisingly, after the pushy crowded streets of London, the soothing open fields of the Emerald Isle were all the excitement Richard seemed to want. Clearly, London was not his 'cup of tea' any more. I made jokes about it saying, "London was so last year," but later, after the diagnosis, it saddened me greatly to think that a city that had brought Richard so much adventure and satisfaction in his twenties was now a destination he could no longer cope with and was somewhere to which he would never return.

In Ireland, everything came more easily to him. Memory, conversations and decision making improved and with that a level of his former confidence resurfaced. His anxiety decreased, facial expressions softened, eyes sparkled and he laughed freely.

The cottage we were staying in had a large back yard with a beautiful view of village houses, a church spire and woolly flocks grazing on distant hills. Richard frequently wandered out to the garden admiring the scenery and the peaceful steady environment. The world he occupied had slowed down. It was now travelling at his pace.

We all had such a wonderful week in Ireland it lulled us all into a false sense of security. When it came time for Richard and I to leave for Portugal ahead of the others we assured them that we could manage. Trying to block out memories of London I kept saying to myself, "How hard is it after all, just to get on a plane?" I actually already knew the answer but this time I would be super vigilant and stay on red alert.

Our tickets had been booked twelve months in advance and at that time I wasn't aware that Richard would be struggling so much to keep up. This trip had really highlighted that it wasn't just normal stress he was experiencing. I planned to try and persuade him to go to the doctor on our return to Adelaide, although I was even beginning to wonder what parts of the holiday he would actually remember.

Our flight to Lisbon was smooth and delightfully uneventful. I wondered if everyone else knew that boredom could feel so good. On arrival we checked in to a charming family-operated hotel adjacent to the impressive Avenida da Liberdade. We were both in high spirits. After our recuperation in Ireland we appeared to be 'all-systems go!' and set off on foot to soak up the vibrant boulevard atmosphere and explore the city sights. We drifted past smart hotels, historic monuments and admired the upmarket shops. We had dinner in an open-air café under the stars and it felt as if the world we used to know was welcoming us back. The day was topped off with a delicious complimentary glass of white port in our elegant hotel lounge. A perfect end to a perfect day.

During the next few days we were fortunate enough to be escorted around Lisbon by a friend of Richard's from his early Port Lincoln days who was now a resident there. We toured the historic Mosteiro dos Jeronimos and the Torre di Belem and ate more heavenly tasting custard tarts than I care to remember. We had such a wonderful time that we felt reluctant to leave but our journey to Sintra beckoned and we were back to being on our own. Again I asked myself, "How hard can it be? All you have to do is get Richard and the luggage on to a train, for heaven's sake. Sintra is only about forty-five minutes out of Lisbon. You will have an amazing experience when you get there."

Yet again I was proved to be just a tad too optimistic.

On the train ride, the sky became overcast and started to pour. To say the heavens had burst a leak was not an exaggeration. Growing up in South Australia, which is one of the driest states on the driest continent on earth, I had never seen such a wall of water in my life. The deluge was still going when we pulled into the station and it showed no signs of stopping.

We investigated the taxi situation but just stepping onto the curb to hail one meant we would be instantly drenched and our luggage too. This was not an appealing prospect so we went back into the station and I checked out suitable places to wait out the storm.

Richard was starting to get quite agitated now so I had to think fast. I had never seen him like that before but there was no time to dwell on it. My brain was in over-drive. A quick solution was needed here. I would think about it when we were safe and warm and dry and enjoying the company of our travelling companions again. They were driving up from Lisbon and due to arrive at the cottage where we were all staying sometime before midnight. I was fairly sure there wouldn't be any provisions there and nothing would be open in the village by the time we arrived. All I could think of was that if Richard had a good meal and a glass of wine that might help relax him a little or at the very least distract him until I had a chance to come up with Plan B.

Being a local station, there wasn't a lot of choice in eating places but I found a nice little typical Portuguese café opposite a Pizza

Hut. The cafe looked warm and welcoming and some of the signs were in English. The staff smiled at us and invited us to come in. "Come on, this will be fun," I said "let's try out some local food and maybe one of those special custard tarts you like."

To my great surprise, Richard flatly refused to go in. I was stunned. He stood there immovably like a giant six-foot pillar of stone. No amount of coaxing worked. He wanted Pizza Hut or nothing. I glanced towards the station entrance and it was still bucketing down. 'Nothing' was not an option so in we went. He was so out of character by now that I had no clue where this was going. He wasn't interested in anything fancy or even any of the varieties of pizza toppings he would normally choose at home. He wanted a cheese pizza and Coke and that was it. I helped him place the order. Situation now semi under control.

Richard munched on the pizza slowly as the rain continued. I just stared out the window at the real Portugal that we were totally ignoring. Aside from the rain, we could have been anywhere, even at home.

Eventually the rain eased a little and after being rejected by three taxis I finally found a driver who could understand the address of the cottage, written down on a soggy piece of paper. Hooray, rescued at last!

The drive to the village took twenty-five minutes, which gave me time to reflect. This was like the Café Royal scenario all over again. Richard had gravitated towards the familiar. When there was too much unfamiliarity for him to process his agitation, shut-down started.

Then it suddenly dawned on me. I had taken Richard out of our home environment, thinking it would be wonderfully refreshing. It had just the opposite effect. Whatever was ailing Richard was now out in the open. He had been able to mask it reasonably well at home and pass it off as tiredness and business stress but not any more. This holiday had totally blown his cover. There was no more hiding, something was definitely wrong.

When we arrived home, I organised a doctor's appointment and then a referral to a specialist in memory disorders for a full evaluation. Many tests later, our rising fears were confirmed.

TAKE-AWAYS

CHAPTER 3

- Travel (particularly overseas) can disorientate people with Alzheimer's

- Travel light. Take only one piece of carry-on luggage, preferably with a shoulder strap

- Keep your passports in your own hand, look after the money, the tickets, travel documents

- Going through airport security is difficult because it is not part of long-term memory

- Where possible choose seats at the rear of the plane which only has two seats in the row

- Toilet doors on planes are challenging and everything in the toilet is unfamiliar e.g. tap, flush button, lock on door

- Meal and snack trays can prove difficult with lots of little containers to open

- Pack some calming items for use in the cabin such as favourite books or music

Chapter 4

THE BLACK SUITCASE

Travelling locally

> "The art of being happy lies in the power of extracting
> happiness from common things."
>
> *Henry Ward Beecher*

These days suitcases come in many different shapes and sizes and a variety of colours and patterns but have you ever noticed that when you are standing in front of the luggage carousel waiting for your suitcase to magically appear that the majority seem to be black? I hadn't given it much thought until one such non-descript black bag became an instrument of unwarranted chaos in my life.

Richard had been diagnosed with younger onset Alzheimer's for a few years when some friends who lived in Port Lincoln (about a one-hour flight from Adelaide) offered to entertain and look after him for the weekend so that he could have some fun and Jack and I could have some respite. Everyone was excited by this prospect.

Richard was looking forward to going back to his hometown and catching up with his old friends, we were happy for him and also unashamedly looking forward to a much needed break from the 24/7 caring routine. It was definitely a win-win for everyone.

On Friday night while we drove to the airport we joked and laughed about all the adventures that lay ahead of him. The weekend activities were starting off 'full throttle' with a sell-out concert at the Port Lincoln Nautilus Arts Centre featuring, among other things, an Elvis tribute. Richard joked that there would be 'dancing in the aisles' and he was going to 'rock around the clock.' It was lovely to see him so excited and animated. A lot of Elvis's hits were still stored in Richard's long-term memory and he could still remember most of the words. This clearly gave him pleasure and a little of the confidence and sparkle of the pre-Alzheimer's Richard returned during his enthusiastic rendition of "Blue Suede Shoes."

On arrival, Richard was feeling so buoyed up he asked just to be left at the drop-off zone. He was pretty convincing and his behaviour in the car had seemed so normal that I almost fell for it. I hesitated for a second and then decided to err on the side of caution and said, "No, that's all right Darling, I have plenty of time, I'll park the car and walk in with you." Inside the terminal, Richard assured me for the second time that he would be fine to catch the plane without assistance, although now confronted by the buzz and activity inside the airport his confidence seemed to have slipped a little.

Jollying him along I said, "Well I've come this far, I might as well go all the way to the gate with you." A look of relief and a big smile spread across his face. I discretely handed Richard over to the flight attendant and whispered that he might need a little extra assistance because he had 'a brain injury.' It was inaccurate but it was the best explanation I could think of at the time. She was very busy with a queue of other passengers but she winked her acknowledgement and I gave Richard a big hug and a kiss and waved him goodbye as he was escorted down the ramp. He was so healthy looking and well-groomed that no-one would have believed that he might need extra help and Alzheimer's would be the last thing that they would think of.

I felt elated when I got into my car. We had actually done something normal and carried it off without a hitch. Our friends would be there to meet Richard at the other end and he was all set for a wonderful weekend. Although they hadn't seen Richard for a few years they assured me that they would take excellent care of him and provide assistance whenever he needed it. I was thrilled by their generosity and unselfishness.

At home I settled down on our comfiest sofa with a blanket and a glass of wine all set for a relaxing night in front of the TV until Jack got home to make our weekend plans. It was barely fifteen minutes until the phone rang.

"Hello, is that Mrs Cranwell?"

"Yes," I said tentatively, thinking it was very late for a telemarketer or a charity call.

"It's the manager from the Port Lincoln Airport here. I have your suitcase and it's getting late….. the terminal is empty…..I need to close up the airport for the night so that the staff can go home…. there is an elderly lady here with me and her bag is missing."

"There must be some mistake," I mumbled.

"No, I'm sure there isn't," he assured me and then went on to describe in punishing detail the black suitcase with the green name tag and my contact details on it. I was stunned into silence.

"The lady is getting pretty anxious and upset over here…..the case has got her medication in it and she has to take it tonight or she'll get really sick," he said.

"Oh my God," I thought, some poor lady could wind up in the Port Lincoln Hospital because Richard or his friends has picked up the wrong bag from the luggage trolley. Could it get any worse, I wondered?

Apparently so.....

I hung up quickly, promising the manager I would contact Richard's friends and arrange the transfer as soon as possible. This was good in theory but proved a lot harder in implementation.

Option 1

Understandably, our friends would have turned off their mobile phones but even if they were on it is unlikely that they could be heard over the sound of five hundred excited baby boomers grooving to the sound of Elvis reincarnated belting out "Shake, Rattle and Roll." So I drew a blank there.

Option 2

Next I try the concert venue. "The Arts Centre office is closed... ..."Please call back between nine am and five pm from Monday to Friday." Helpful?...not really.

Option 3

Of course there are venue staff on duty but they are out on the floor and I have no way of knowing their mobile numbers. No joy there.

Meanwhile, the airport manager calls me back to check on progress. I have nothing positive. Clearly he is feeling the increasing pressure from his staff and the unfortunate passenger. I assure him I will keep on task and will phone back as soon as I have made a breakthrough. However, I am fast running out of options.

At this point our respite weekend is proving more stressful than a normal weekend. I thought, "If this is what respite is like, we might need to reconsider next time." I look at my watch and time is marching on. I have a sudden vision of an ambulance on its way to the Port Lincoln Airport to rescue the distraught passenger.

Option 4

I send a few more text messages and leave a few more voicemails. How many is too many I wonder? Surely, they can't go unnoticed for much longer. It seems an eternity since I left the first message. What's wrong with these people? Why aren't they checking their phones constantly? How dare they be so blissfully ignorant of the crisis that has unfolded tonight?

Nothing for it now. All strategies and frantic activity have failed. I put my emergency management training into good practice and escalate the incident.

I call the Port Lincoln Police Station and explain the unfortunate situation to the very patient and kindly duty officer. He listens intently. Is it because he can't get a word in or his experience in handling hysterical people late at night?

We are in luck. The officer advises me that it is a quiet night (for crime) in Port Lincoln. "All the rowdy ones are at the concert," he assures me. The concert hall is only a few minutes walk from the station. He can lock the station (it's not as if anyone is likely to break in to a police station) and stroll down to the venue and ask the staff to make an announcement during a break in the performance. Is this the breakthrough?

So somewhere between song brackets our friends in the audience are alerted to come to the foyer and meet the policeman. And several phone calls later in a scene reminiscent of a Check-Point Charlie prisoner exchange in Cold War Berlin, the exchange takes place. Two identical looking black bags are swapped in the town jetty car park. A few minutes later I receive a text to say, "The eagle has landed! "The situation is under control and all are safe." Breathing collective sighs of relief I reach for my wine and Jack his cola. I think we have earned it. Respite re-started.

Richard had a wonderful weekend and was spoilt rotten by his friends. They organised a barbeque and invited half a dozen of his former business and sporting mates to come around and spend time with him - a wonderful idea. Jack had a pleasant weekend catching up with his friends and I deepened my relationship with the sofa and the television remote control.

On the Monday, Richard travelled back to Adelaide by car with an old friend who had appointments in the city. That night we welcomed him home at the front door. He was tired and happy. The weekend had been a great success but I can't help glare at the mischievous black suitcase sitting innocently by the doorstep. It immediately went into early retirement in the big cupboard under the stairs, not to see the light of day again for many years to come.

TAKE-AWAYS

CHAPTER 4

- Beware of that look of old confidence - it doesn't necessarily mean renewed competence

- Responsibility for luggage or any carry-on items is challenging

- It is difficult to process surroundings with too much activity happening

- Where possible, wear coats and jackets until on the plane to avoid carrying them

- Pack everything else in checked luggage

- Aim for the carer to be the only one responsible for anything you wish to take on board

Chapter 5

SOCIAL LEPROSY

Loneliness and the Stigma Factor

> "When we are no longer able to change a situation – we are
> challenged to change ourselves."
>
> *Viktor E. Frankl*

Fame is fleeting or so they say, but when Richard developed Alzheimer's we discovered that some friendships can be like that too. It was as if we had sprayed ourselves from head to toe in tropical strength bug repellent, only instead of repelling insects we were repelling friends we had known for years. This phenomenon came on subtly at first and with everything else going on in our lives it took a little while to notice that a pattern was emerging.

One of the most telling signs was that the phone was not ringing quite so often and that Saturday night social invitations seemed to be drying up. We had previously enjoyed a reasonably active social life and the realisation was slowly beginning to sink in. Sometimes we would hear on the grape vine of weekend gatherings that we would normally be invited to went by without us.

The hardest part was in the early days of his illness when Richard still had some awareness about what was going on. "I wonder why I haven't heard from Tim and Jane in a while," he would say. "Perhaps they are overseas," I would suggest, hoping this would counter his feelings of rejection. That strategy was sometimes successful but deep down I believe in the early days, post diagnosis, he knew what was going on - his 'mates' were avoiding him because of the nature of his illness. It was just too confronting for them. The only reason I have ever been grateful for Alzheimer's was knowing that eventually the memory of this hurt would fade for him.

Often I would bump into friends or acquaintances at the local shopping centre or in the city. They would tell me they had heard Richard wasn't well and politely enquire after his health. What most surprised me was the tone and manner in which questions were framed - as if Richard had contracted something temporary like a virus or the flu and that there was a presumption that someone as young and seemingly healthy as he was would recover. It wasn't hard to recognise what was going on here. They were experiencing denial, just like we had.

Some were genuinely interested in knowing more about Alzheimer's and would enquire further. I would try and answer their questions as precisely and simply as possible and give examples of the sorts of difficulties Richard was experiencing: such as he was no longer able to drive and that I had to take the car and house keys away from him. Other examples included his need for assistance with bathing, shaving and dressing or the fact that I had to confiscate his wallet because he was no longer able to handle financial transactions of any kind. Even purchasing something in a shop was beyond him. Cash might as well have been Monopoly 'money' for all Richard knew. I also removed his lovely watch that was his 40th birthday gift from me and put it in a drawer to pass on to Jack at a later date. If I was asked what Richard did during the day to occupy his time now that he no longer was able to work I did not hide the fact that he attended a dementia day centre Monday to Friday while I was at work. I always said what a wonderful support it was to Richard and our family.

It was usually at this precise moment when talking to men of Richard's age that I noticed their eyes would start to glaze over and the rising fear for their own mortality would descend on their faces like crimson velvet curtains on a West End theatre stage. "Oh My God, if that happened to Dick Cranwell, it could happen to anyone, it could even happen to me" was written all over their faces. If this had only happened once I would not be writing about it now but this happened quite often to the extent that while engaging in conversation I wondered, how long until 'curtain-fall' this time?

It was not that I had dramatised the situation, in fact I went to particular care to impart this news gently because I was fully aware of the shock reaction it would create. Richard had been such a healthy man and a great amateur sportsman in his youth that it made his illness totally incomprehensible to some. Richard attending a dementia day centre? They just could not get their heads around it.

One of the most disappointing and bitter pills I had to swallow came after Richard had moved into the nursing home. A chance meeting with a colleague of Richard's had resulted in the usual conversation with the usual enquiries. It was all going fine but suddenly turned sour when the gentleman looked me directly in the face and said, "Of course I would love to visit Richard but I don't do hospitals.....I am not very good at them." This took my breath away. It was a rare moment of speechlessness for me. Apart from the fact that Richard was at this time now in a care facility and not a hospital made no difference whatsoever. It was just as insulting and selfish, regardless of the type of institution where Richard was living.

For me, one of the saddest aspects of this story is that, in his heyday, Richard was the sort of man who was well known for his kindness, generosity and nobility of spirit. He did not put his own needs above the needs of others and ironically he often responded to frailty and signs of dementia in others. For example, one of the regular customers in Richard's business was a charming elderly gentleman who was well into his eighties. He came in every week on the same day to buy his lottery ticket. Richard always went out of his way to acknowledge this gentleman and have a chat with him because he was aware that he was lonely and that his weekly trip to the shopping mall was the highlight of his week.

One day a relative came in to the shop and bought the ticket on behalf of the old man because he was ill. On hearing this Richard said, "Don't worry about that, I will take it round to him personally." He promptly left the business, taking the ticket with him and another complimentary ticket and drove twenty minutes to the old man's house and visited with him for nearly an hour. Another time a lady came into our store. Richard recognised the lady as the mother of one of his business competitors from a near-by shopping centre. Richard telephoned the lady's son and said, "I think there is something you ought to know. Your mother has been into my business. I think she is having problems with money because when she purchases something she brings the item to the cash register and opens up her purse for the staff to take the right amount of money out. If she is doing that in my shop she is possibly doing it in others. My staff are all extremely honest and trustworthy but I can't vouch for all the other businesses around town."

In early 2005, two years after Richard had been diagnosed with Alzheimer's, we went on an island holiday off the coast of Far North Queensland. Overseas holidays had been abandoned for somewhere closer to home. Calm blue skies, the crystal clear blue-green waters of the Great Barrier Reef and delicious food and wine all contributed to a delightful escape from winter in Adelaide. All went pretty well. We swam and sunbathed and went on lovely peaceful walks around the island. After seven beautiful days we returned to Adelaide looking refreshed and sporting lightly golden suntans. I returned to work on Monday and a few days later flew off to Canberra to attend a two-day government meeting.

It was during the second session, just before lunch on the first day, that I received a frantic phone call from Ainslie. Richard had had a heart attack at work and been resuscitated by the paramedics in the ambulance. She had just been notified and was on her way to the hospital. I took the first flight back and went straight to the hospital. Richard spent ten days in hospital and then three weeks in a special rehabilitation hospital.

News of Richard's heart attack spread like wildfire throughout our circle of friends and acquaintances. Then a most unusual thing happened that was totally unexpected. All of a sudden the phone started ringing again with people wanting to express their concern and pass on their well wishes to Richard. Nearly every day I received two or three calls. I was pleased of course by this increase in concern for Richard's wellbeing but I was baffled. I couldn't work out what was going on. We had never experienced anything like this level of concern or enquiry the whole time Richard had been diagnosed with Alzheimer's and exactly the same groups of people were involved.

Then of course it dawned on me. The concept of a heart attack was something people were familiar with and something they could get their heads around. They knew what questions to ask. They could talk about surgery and stents and drugs and their voices didn't falter and their words didn't flounder. The topic was familiar and 'safe' and though still upsetting it was nowhere near as confronting as dementia. "Oh, I get it," I thought. "A heart attack for men is like breast cancer for women. Everyone knows about it. The information is right out in the open which minimises the mystery and the stigma."

One particular circle of friends that did continue to make Richard and I still welcome after he was diagnosed with Alzheimer's consisted of my close school girlfriends and their husbands and another couple, Jill and Tony. If it wasn't for this small group of friends who supported us during those years before Richard went into residential care, our social life would have been almost non-existent. We were invited to their homes for barbeques and dinner parties and were often included in their circle when they went out to dinner.

Sometimes when we were in restaurants, Richard would forget which wine glass he was drinking from and he would start drinking from the glass of the person next to him. No one made a fuss. They just politely guided his hand back to his own glass or asked for another glass from the waiter for themselves. Chinese banquets were a little more challenging. I remember one evening we were all seated at a round table. We had ordered a banquet with about eight different courses. Everything was going well and we were all having a great time. Richard wasn't leading any conversations but he was right in the thick of it and enjoying the friendly banter. He was laughing and smiling and I could see he felt included around the table and most importantly relevant.

The waitress brought two over-flowing platters of appetisers to be shared within the group. There was a beautiful selection of piping hot spring rolls, peanut chicken satays, pork steamed dumplings with soy sauce and large crispy prawn crackers. One of the platters was placed right in front of me. That was handy so I organised Richard's plate and got him started. I knew he would struggle with decision making and coordinating the use of tongs let alone chopsticks to select individual pieces. For Richard to make his own selections while someone else was holding a platter in front of him just created too much pressure for him. That would have been too many thoughts and too many actions for him to process in such a short time and in a busy noisy restaurant.

We all enjoyed our appetisers and then a steady flow of main dishes arrived. We circulated the dishes to be shared around the table and when a dish landed in front of Richard I helped him again. We still had a few more main courses to arrive but I think everyone had taken the edge off their appetites. This was a good thing and very timely as it turned out.

When I was inevitably distracted by conversation Richard started digging into a plate of chicken and cashew nuts, one of his favourites, and had nearly devoured the lot. "What's wrong with this picture?" I suddenly thought, "Oops! We are meant to be sharing each course." He was totally oblivious to the fact that he was supposed to take a little and then pass the plate on.

This is how he now processed information - in short bursts.... Someone had given him food......he was eating the food....perfectly logical to someone with short-term memory loss. My friend Anne had observed what had happened and she just smiled at me and said, "Don't worry. No one else has even noticed what is going on. Richard has done us all a favour. There are still a few more dishes yet to be served and we are all getting very full anyway." I still felt a little uncomfortable and so when it came time to pay the bill I explained and offered to pay extra but everyone was very kind and told me not to be so silly.

As Richard's illness progressed, the logistics of social events like that became increasingly more difficult so we started to spend more time at home. It wasn't a conscious decision but something that just gradually evolved. Unfamiliar places that were not part of what remained of Richard's long-term memory were just too much of an obstacle. For instance, unless we had another couple with us and the husband could show Richard to the men's bathroom, wait for him and escort him back to our table, it always became a worry. One time Richard was invited to watch a cricket game at the Adelaide Oval. Typical of such large venues, there were two doors into the men's toilets. Both the doorways were at opposite ends of the bathroom and looked identical. When he exited, Richard chose the opposite one from the direction in which he had come and headed off in the wrong direction. He was missing-in-action for the next thirty minutes, causing his hosts great concern, although fortunately he was not too aware of his predicament.

For me it was apparent that my life as a carer had radically changed but for our friends and associates, life went on as normal.

Luckily, a few old friends, Rob, Mick and John (who, like Richard, all had rural upbringings) and Bernie his volunteer carer, were able to conquer their own fears and overlook Richard's memory difficulties. They could see past the stigma associated with dementia. True, their friend of many years was altered but he was still there inside and they reached out to him just as they knew he would have done for them.....without a moment's hesitation.

TAKE-AWAYS

CHAPTER 5

- The carer gradually loses their spouse, best friend and companion

- The loneliness and isolation the person with Alzheimer's experiences also impacts on their carer

- Carers often spend so much time in their caring and domestic roles that there is not so much time, energy or money to socialise

- There is little time for carer hobbies which adds to the sense of isolation

- Loneliness is not an easy thing to admit to oneself or to other people

- You will find out who are really your true friends and who are not

Chapter 6

WHO MOVED MY STREET?

Time to stop driving

> "If we can learn to accept early on that life is going to be a mixed bag of positive and negative experiences, we're going to be much better equipped to deal with whatever life will inevitably throw at us down the track."
>
> *Matthew Johnstone*

One of my fondest memories of my father was when he told me stories about his adventures while travelling with my mother. Sometimes when they stopped in a city or town my parents would split up for a short while to indulge my mother's need for some 'retail therapy' and give Dad some freedom to undertake reconnaissance and find a suitable restaurant for lunch or dinner. Dad would give Mum clear directions on how to find him. He would arrive early at the well chosen landmark and almost without fail watch my mother approach from the opposite direction from which he had told her to return. Apparently she would just smile, laugh and shrug her shoulders and say, "Oh well, someone moved the street."

It is therefore not surprising that I inherited my mother's haphazard sense of direction and occasional desire to turn a map upside down while reading it. Thank goodness I married a man who did not suffer from this affliction. Richard was quite skilled at orienteering and always possessed a keen sense of direction. We rarely ever got lost or took a wrong direction when he was either driver or navigator. Alzheimer's changed all of that.

At the diagnosis in February 2003, the doctor advised us that a person with dementia may still be able to drive safely for some time after the diagnosis. This was very welcome news for both of us. For Richard it was a real confidence booster. Being able to drive meant he could continue to maintain his independence by driving himself to work, pursue hobbies and attend social activities and sometimes take the children to school and weekend sport. For me, it meant we could maintain some normal family functions and routines while still trying to come to terms with the diagnosis and the subtle changes in Richard's cognitive skills.

The dementia specialist referred Richard to a Dementia Driving Clinic for assessment. He undertook his first driving assessment in mid-2003 and was found to be well within the safe driving skill range. We were both delighted with the result and it gave him a real boost in confidence. He had a smile from ear to ear when he got the results. It was the first good news we had received since his diagnosis. We popped some champagne to celebrate when we got home because it was important to recognise his achievement. We both knew it would not always be this way so that made it even more important to seize the day.

Even though Richard frequently misplaced keys and showed other signs of memory loss such as losing track of time, dates and confusion under pressure, he continued to drive safely for nearly three years. However, in early 2005 the deterioration in his memory loss was becoming more pronounced - with heightened frequency and duration. I was starting to feel uncomfortable about Richard having any passengers at all and for the other drivers on the road and I thought it was time to raise my concerns with his doctor on return from our holiday. A few events had raised the alarm.

As mentioned in the previous chapter, I took Richard to Queensland for a holiday in 2005. We had stayed in the resort before in 1997 and we had both really enjoyed ourselves. I thought this would be a far easier holiday than going overseas. No need to worry about long haul flights, passports, foreign languages or currency. There was only one resort on the island so I thought Richard could wander at leisure and enjoy the freedom of exploring the small island with no fear of him getting lost for either of us.

I had especially requested a room adjacent to the undercover stairwell so that the stairs would be easy to find if he was on his own. We were on an upper floor so that we could capture views of the oasis sized swimming pool below and look out across the pristine beach to the crystal clear blue-green waters lapping the neighbouring island. "This will be so relaxing," I thought. "Richard loved it here before and he will love it again, I am sure. After we have been swimming, if he gets restless he can go down the stairs for another swim and I can wave to him from the balcony or he can go off and explore the beautifully maintained tropical gardens and greenhouses." This plan was good in theory but it backfired miserably on us right at the start.

When I made the reservation I was so focussed on getting a room near the stairs and the freedom the resort grounds would give Richard, that I had overlooked one small detail that would change everything. The resort was built with all the rooms facing the beautiful sea view. Guests enter rooms from an impeccably decorated and maintained rear veranda. The doorway to each room was recessed from the veranda to create a sense of entry and the room number was displayed on a discrete brass plaque. Therein lay the problem. When you looked all the way down the long veranda, the doorway to every room was identical and the only distinguishing feature was the little brass plaque with the four-digit room number.

For someone suffering memory loss this was an unexpected and challenging hurdle. I had chosen an end room away from the lift well, thinking that operating the lifts might be a bit confusing for Richard. Our room was located on the third floor which I thought would also be easy for Richard to remember (i.e. three blind mice, three wise men). We had the closest room to the stairwell and it exited right next to the swimming pool.

However, it didn't matter which floor you exited the stairwell from, every long veranda looked exactly the same. Unless you could remember your floor level and room number you were guaranteed to get plenty of exercise walking backwards and forwards to reception (if you could remember where that was) to get your room details written down for you.

On the first day, Richard was feeling confident and he was keen to go off exploring on his own. I thought he would only be about five minutes but when he wasn't back in twenty I started to become concerned and I set out to find him. I walked out into the passageway and fortunately, because all the rooms on all three levels opened onto verandas, I was able to run along each veranda calling out his name. Eventually I got an answer from the floor below and we were reunited. I could see Richard was starting to get distressed so I made a joke as a circuit breaker. I teased him about the fact that he was wearing me out by playing a game of 'hide and seek' with me. We both had a hearty laugh but after that incident Richard never left my side for the remaining six days of our holiday. We still enjoyed ourselves swimming, walking, playing putt-putt golf, having cocktails at sunset and delicious food but on our plane flight home, nothing could compensate me for the realisation that Richard's freedom to roam at will, even in a fairly confined environment, was quietly slipping away.

I resolved to contact the doctor before the end of that week but it was a few days after we returned home that Richard had a heart attack. This brought into focus the need to solve the issue of driving. After the time in hospital he was also very keen to demonstrate his fitness to resume normal activities and was disheartened when I told him the doctor had advised me at the hospital that he would not be able to drive again for six months after his heart attack.

Even though he was learning to accept limitations that were creeping into his life it was still a frustrating time for Richard and the rest of us. We managed by choosing activities for Richard closer to home and a few friends and extended family helped out with daytime activities and transportation. As the months went by, Richard's cognitive skills seemed to deteriorate at a slightly more rapid pace than before. We weren't sure if this was related to the heart attack or another stage in the Alzheimer's disease process. While still not able to work or drive, boredom was becoming an issue that really needed to be resolved.

A special dementia day centre for people aged sixty and above provided the solution.

Richard was very reluctant at first but eventually came to accept that he was moving out of the mainstream workforce. He seemed to have some awareness that working in our business was becoming more and more stressful and getting beyond him. I was also aware that his presence was creating difficulties for the staff and we were all very relieved by his gradual acceptance of taking a few days out of the business each week. Perhaps my description of his reduced hours as 'preparing for retirement' rather than 'full retirement' helped eased the transition - but I am not sure.

However, reduced hours in the business is one thing but not being able to drive is another matter entirely. To Richard, continuation of driving symbolised his independence and freedom. He had sufficient awareness at this time to know that stopping driving would hasten his dependence on others and increase his sense of general frustration and isolation from friends, family and business colleagues.

It was at about the four-month mark in Richard's recovery from the heart attack that I discovered that the time recommended to wait before recommencing driving after a heart attack was actually six weeks, not six months. Looking back now I realise I was very stressed so I probably had not taken in all of the details of the doctor's instructions very clearly when Richard was sent home. All I knew was that it was a very serious condition and that compounded with younger onset Alzheimer's, six months rest from normal activities made sense to me.

I genuinely believed six months rest was the requirement but Richard was becoming more and more restless and there was pressure from other family members for him to recommence driving so I agreed to take him to the doctor and discuss the issue with her. The doctor explained my mistake and that the normal waiting time to recommence driving after a heart attack was indeed actually six weeks and not six months. I was indeed "the bad guy." My mistake, albeit genuine, had delayed Richard's return to his previous lifestyle and activities by four months. Listening to the doctor, I felt a mixture of guilt and a niggling doubt at the same time. I felt guilty that I had deprived Richard of his liberty but I also wondered whether my mistake had been a blessing in disguise that had possibly saved lives. Of course, there was no way of knowing but deep down my inner voice was telling me that Richard's driving days were already in the past and attempting to revive them now was indeed just tempting fate.

There was only one way to find out.

The doctor agreed to refer Richard back for another special driving assessment but warned him that this time he might find the test tougher and even if he did pass it might be time to consider relinquishing his licence. Richard nodded several times in agreement but I recognised his resolute expression. There is nothing quite as obvious as raw determination. Clearly, the thought of losing his licence was totally repugnant to him but I had heard the doctor's warning and knew that she was trying to prepare him for the inevitable. I was also grateful for her explanation because I would not have to be 'the bad guy' again, or so I thought. It would be the doctor and staff at the dementia driving clinic whose role it would be to break the bad news to Richard. They were trained for this role - I was not.

The clinic was busy so we had to wait over three weeks for the appointment. However, about a week and a half before Richard was due to take the driving test I had confirmation that his driving days were drawing to a close.

We had moved into our new home just before Richard's diagnosis so the design and layout was never stored in his long term memory. The house was long and narrow, built on three levels and had three bathrooms. When we first moved in, it wasn't something that was immediately obvious but Richard's temperament was beginning to change. At certain times of the day he was uncharacteristically impatient and looked stressed. I asked him if he wanted anything to eat or drink or needed to go to the bathroom. He always said he was fine but then would start wandering around the house going in and out of rooms and up and down the stairs several times. At first I thought he was just moving away from the kitchen or television noise but after a while his expression and body language made me wonder if he was beginning to have difficulty finding the bathroom.

Then one day we were in the middle of our bedroom about to go downstairs and Richard asked me, "Where is the bathroom?" "Oh dear," I thought, "we are really in trouble now....someone has 'moved' the bathroom." Only it wasn't funny at all. What made matters worse was the fact that the closest bathroom to where we were standing was the en-suite to the bedroom. It was 2.5 metres away and Richard used it every day.

As the day for the driving test approached I couldn't help but ask myself, "If someone can't find an attached bathroom, surely they should not be driving any more?"

It is worth noting here that observation of behaviour changes is often only obvious to the primary carer because these changes can occur at different times and on different days. Also, the primary carer has usually supervised and/or assisted with bathing, dressing and grooming. These daily processes usually remain unseen by other family members and friends giving them an ill-informed opinion of the level of support the person with Alzheimer's requires because their diminishing skills are 'hidden' from view. The person's appearance when they are bathed, groomed and dressed can be 'deceptively' normal.

In our case, when Richard caught up with extended family and friends he looked exactly the same as he always did. Nothing in his physical appearance (until later stages) had changed. He smelt clean, he was shaved, his hair was washed and brushed and he wore neat and tidy fashionable clothes as he had always done. This led most people to believe, in fact expect, that Richard could look after himself and that he was able to function the same as he always had, apart from a little forgetfulness. Had they seen him standing in the middle of the bedroom looking for the en-suite bathroom they would have begun to realise his true situation.

Richard had not driven since his heart attack and was getting anxious about his forthcoming driving test. He mentioned this to a friend that he saw on a weekly basis. They offered to take him out for driving and parking practice in a vacant supermarket car-park the night before his test. I would not have supported the idea had I been informed. In my view, anyone who becomes agitated and confused because they cannot find their way around their own home is going to have difficulty driving independently and may be putting themselves and other road users at risk.

It was just giving him false hope. This may sound harsh but day to day care best acquaints you with the subtle changes in cognitive decline. Denial is common amongst friends and family. They want the person with Alzheimer's to continue functioning as they normally would because they cannot stand the thought that their loved one is slipping away. However, it is impossible to maintain the status quo when you are standing on 'uneven' ground.

The next day we left home early to arrive at the driving clinic in time for Richard to relax before his test. The receptionist gave us a lovely warm and calming greeting when we arrived. She could see that it wasn't just Richard who was nervous. There was a lot riding on these test results. We didn't have to wait long before he was given a briefing by the driving instructor. Suddenly they were off!

After what seemed like an eternity (but was probably only about forty-five minutes) they returned and we were asked to wait while his assessment was considered. Our nerves were frayed so I read Richard a magazine article to fill in the time. Finally we were summoned and off we trouped into the boardroom like a pair of unrepentant heretics ready to face the Spanish Inquisition.

From recollection, the informal panel consisted of a neuropsychologist, the driving instructor and a research student. Well, if the driving test hadn't done it already, the effort involved in meeting so many strangers in a formal setting was enough to make Richard look pale and exhausted. He appeared to struggle with every introduction and when words totally failed him, he simply nodded his head in acknowledgement.

Introductions and pleasantries were out of the way and then it was down to business. Firstly, the neuropsychologist, who led the discussion, prefaced his remarks by explaining that their collective responsibility was to ensure that everyone who passed this special driving assessment was a safe driver and indeed fit to hold a driving licence. Points were allocated out of a maximum score of one hundred and the pass mark was seventy. The more serious the breach of the road traffic rules, the more points were deducted. One by one the examiners gave their comments.

It all sounded fair and logical but when the neuropsychologist came to sum up and give the final verdict I could feel the axe rising as he spoke. Richard's driving infringements varied in severity but included things like not complying with speed limits, not checking his rear or side mirrors before changing lanes and pulling out from the curb without using the indicator. The most serious issue however was his inability to anticipate what other drivers might be doing or how to take evasive action himself. Apparently, at one stage during the on-road test the instructor had to intervene to prevent an imminent collision!

At this stage of the report Richard looked completely overwhelmed and totally confused. He needed a simple 'yes' or 'no' and for the long ordeal to be over. Despite the empathy and thoughtful explanations, nothing quite prepared us for the result. We sat in stony silence listening intently for any faint sign of hope or face-saving redemption but it was as futile as trying to stop the sun from shining.

We were stunned when Richard's final score was read out loud. He had achieved one of the lowest scores ever recorded at the clinic. Twelve out of a potential one hundred points left everyone in the room momentarily speechless.

We had reached another life changing milestone with absolutely no room for negotiation. Richard's driving days were well and truly over. Understandably, Richard was devastated and vented his anger all the way home. I had never seen him so angry before but fortunately we only lived about five minutes away and somehow I managed to get us home safely.

I am not embarrassed to admit that as our new reality slowly sank in, part of me felt a sense of pure relief that Richard and other road users were no longer at risk from his driving. "Phew, crisis averted," I thought. My judgement had been vindicated by the test results but that was certainly no cause for celebration and I felt terribly sad for him.

But where to from here?

Bewildered doesn't even begin to describe our feelings of loss and uncertainty. Richard's anger took several days to subside. His memory of the driving test had long since evaporated but his emotional response to losing his licence remained acute so I bore the verbal brunt of his disappointment and frustration.

There is no denying it. This was a tough time for everyone in our family. We were all affected. At the time, we had no way of knowing that when Richard lost his licence it solved one concern but opened up many more. We all learnt in no uncertain terms, the true meaning of the phrase describing a situation that 'goes from the frying pan into the fire.'

Richard was still intent on going to his workplace every day. Understandably, the business gave him a sense of purpose, relevance and a reason to get up every morning. He was increasingly losing control of so many aspects of his life and so the business took on even greater importance. It gave him a reference point and his sense of identity as a businessman.

We had not yet resolved what to do when a few days later Richard surprisingly took matters into his own hands. I was at work one morning when I received a frantic phone call from Ainslie. "Mum, Dad's disappeared. I went upstairs and I couldn't find him. I've been driving around the neighbourhood for an hour now and I can't find him anywhere. What should I do? Shall I call the police?"

I left work in such a hurry I don't even remember which route I took home but just as I approached our driveway I received a call from Sherree, our business manager. Richard had arrived safely but unexpectedly at the business and she was just checking to see if I was aware of his movements.

Ainslie and I breathed a huge sigh of relief and as our nerves started to recover we realised what an extraordinary thing had happened. Richard had walked to the next street and caught an express bus that went all the way through the city and down to our business, a journey of approximately sixty minutes. If he could manage that on his own without any coaching then we had a possible solution to our transport issues, for a while at least. I couldn't help but smile with pride at his courage and determination.

I drove Richard to the bus stop the next morning and waited until I saw him get safely on the bus. This method of transport worked quite well for a few weeks until one day Richard got off the bus in the city and got lost. He hadn't wandered too far from the bus stop but streets that had been familiar all his life were suddenly no longer recognisable. As chance would have it, out of all the people in the city that day, Richard bumped into Sherree's boyfriend Wayne, who had worked with disabled people for many years. He had known Richard for over a decade and it didn't take him long to figure out what had happened. He escorted Richard to the bus stop and waited until he was safely on the right bus that would take him directly to his business. Phew, another close call! Maybe the bus wasn't such a great option after all?

The business was a direct link back to Richard's former self and understandably he was going to fight to hang onto it any way he could. Gentle suggestions that maybe he should cut back on his visits to the business were met with outrage and disgust. "It's my business and my life. Stop trying to control me. You can't tell me how to run my life. You are not the boss of me," he said with such force that I found myself unable to respond.

These arrangements couldn't continue but a suitable solution wasn't that easy to find. Richard assured me that he could and would take the bus back and forth to the business without assistance. Remarkably, he managed to do so successfully for several months without a hitch until one day he got off the bus too early again. This time it was halfway between the city and the business. This could have been quite a disastrous event for him because he didn't know the area at all and it would have been a long hot walk to the shopping centre, even for someone who knew the way. Then something quite miraculous happened once again. At the very moment Richard got off the bus and started walking down the street, one of his staff, Viv, walked out to empty her letterbox which was attached to the front fence of her home. After Viv collected her mail she turned around and looked up and could not believe her eyes. There, out of the blue, marching purposely towards her is Richard and a smile breaks out all over his face. "Hello Viv" he says, "good to see you."

Viv realising what had happened took him inside and settled him down with a cup of tea, then phoned ahead to the business. Interestingly, Richard understood he had made a mistake but he begged Viv not to tell anyone. However, I was grateful that she let me in on his latest 'adventure.'

I wasn't at all confident that his luck would hold a third time. Big changes to Richard's routine were now urgently required. A meeting with Richard's specialist was particularly illuminating.

"Richard has reached the stage now where his independence is no longer up to him. You won't be able to look after him and the family on your own. It is too much for one person. You have to get Richard used to other people helping look after him during the daytime at least so that you know he is safe and well cared for." The doctor handed me a general contact phone number for relevant Australian Government health/aged agencies and another for private aged care facilities and warned me that what Richard needed to keep him occupied would not be easy to find. This proved to be very true.

These weren't the sort of phone calls I could make from my workplace. They needed privacy and a great deal of time so I took a day's recreation leave to make the calls from home. It is a day I will never forget as long as I live. I sat at the kitchen table and worked the phone from nine until five. I took thirty minutes off for a lunch break and two bathroom stops. The rest of the time I was either talking or 'on hold.' When I explained our situation, most people I spoke to were empathetic and really wanted to help. The sticking point was Richard's age. He was too young to qualify for any assistance. Every time they entered his details into the computer to assess his eligibility, the results were negative because he was under sixty-five. "How ironic," I thought, "Richard is so young to be getting Alzheimer's but not old enough to access the help he needs."

When it got to 4:45pm my voice was hoarse but I thought I could squeeze in just one more call before all the offices closed for the day. I spoke to a very nice lady who was very supportive but also unable to help with suggestions for Richard's immediate needs. "We really are falling through the cracks," I said and she replied, "I know you want a suitable day program for your husband and I am so sorry I can't help you but would you like me to send you an information book on full-time residential care? You don't require that now but you may need it a bit further down the track." I was so exhausted by this stage that I just said "yes" to show my appreciation for her kind offer and the extra time she had taken to try and help me. Then it occurred to me that it would actually be nice to have something tangible to show for my day's work. I didn't know where we were going to from here or how I was going to solve our problem but at least the book may be helpful in the future.

I went back to work the next day and didn't give the book another thought.

About two weeks later, a parcel arrived in the mail with some brochures and the book. After dinner when Richard had gone to bed I nervously browsed through the information. I dreaded the thought of one day having to admit Richard to a full-time care facility. Reading about it was very confronting but I noticed a few of the facilities had day centres attached that had programs and activities that might be suitable for Richard. I started reading the book more carefully, paying close attention to every listing and advertisement. There just had to be something in that book that could help us. There just had to be!

It was getting late and I was tired, so I almost missed it, but suddenly there it was.......a lifeline in one sentence....."New Day Centre opening, people with dementia aged sixty plus welcome." Finally the answer to all my prayers.... tears flowed freely..... I felt like we had just won the lottery!

This was the only day centre in the whole book that was open to people aged sixty and it was only a fifteen minute drive from our house. We were in the defined catchment zone and fees were partially subsidised by the government. I floated up the stairs to bed that night and slept soundly for the first time in months.

TAKE-AWAYS

CHAPTER 6

- Trust your gut instinct because you are there every single day observing all the subtle little changes of diminishing ability

- When pieced together, all these little "snapshots" form a much larger picture

- You are like a person adding the final touches to a very large complicated jigsaw puzzle

- You have observed these scenes and patterns emerging right from the beginning, therefore you see the whole picture more quickly and clearly than others.

Chapter 7

NEWSFLASH! FULL TIME CARING IS NOT A SPECTATOR SPORT

Avoiding carer burnout and learning to ask for help

> "The secret is in absolutely refusing to let the river beat you down. If I had to, I'd measure my progress in inches. One more inch I've swum – one less inch to swim. Once you know the secret, then nobody's river can bring you down."
>
> *Bette Greene*

Despite the myth, carers are not super human or immortal. It's just convenient for those who prefer someone else to take on the primary caring role and responsibility to think so. Encouraging slaps on the back only go so far and complimentary words such as "Wow.....you are amazing!" "Congratulations you are doing such a great job!" "You should really be proud of yourself" and "I really admire you" wear very thin after a while when they are not backed up by any kind of practical 'concrete' support.

The most common, irritating but perhaps revealing comment of all is, "I don't know how you do it" as if the carer has some magical powers that they can turn on and off when it suits them. This statement also highlights another sharp truth. Spectators don't know how a carer 'does it' because they sometimes intentionally or unintentionally create sufficient space between themselves and the person with Alzheimer's to remain blissfully ignorant of what type or level of assistance is actually required. Spending quality time with this person and their carer will help identify how a carer actually 'does it' and what type or level of support is needed to reduce the pressure on both of them.

What spectators tend to overlook is that many carers have been thrust into the role unexpectedly, without any choice, warning or training. It is a two-edged sword. Carers have to know it is alright asking for help, that asking for help is not a failing and families, friends and neighbours need to appreciate it is not OK to ask vaguely, "Is there anything I can do to help?" Trust me, there will ALWAYS be something you can do to help but it may require a little detective work on your behalf. When you meet the carer and they are reluctant to ask, let a follow-up phone call or a visit guide your contribution. You may never know the exact impact such a small gesture may have on the carer but I can tell you from personal experience it can be huge. Jill used to call me regularly on a Saturday morning and it was an enormous comfort to me knowing I could rely on her phone call. At times it felt like I had been thrown a life buoy. In fact I can even remember times when I used to count the sleeps till Saturday. That's how much those phone calls meant to me, so please never, ever underestimate the impact your gesture may have on the carer.

By mid-2009 my stress level was through the roof. It was only six and a half years since Richard's professional diagnosis but over ten years since he had started showing signs of memory loss.

We were becoming more and more reliant on my full-time salary for living, medical and supplementary caring expenses. Our income from the business had dwindled considerably because we had to employ extra staff to cover Richard's absence and we found ourselves in that unwelcome position of 'expenses up and income down.' This was particularly hard to manage emotionally. I tried to hide my fear from Richard so as not to worry him or let him think I was implying any weakening on his behalf. Part of me knew that he may not realise what our real situation was like but just because his memory was affected did not mean that he was not capable of reading my emotions and the more rattled I looked the more unsettled he became. 'Steady as she goes,' no matter how difficult that was to portray at times, was preferable to watching Richard's anxiety rising, any day.

NAVIGATING ALZHEIMER'S

Day-to-day finances were just one of many issues our family was facing. Richard's memory loss had increased to the level where he was becoming totally dependent on other people for his daily survival. He needed assistance with bathing, grooming, dressing and eating. He was unable to figure out how to turn the taps on in the shower or that once he got out of the shower, that the taps did not turn themselves off. He had not been able to work in the business or drive a car for some time. He could not answer or dial a telephone or be responsible for house keys, a wallet or his watch. Whenever he left the house with a carer to take him to the day centre the only possessions he had on him were the clothes he was wearing. He could not boil the kettle, make a piece of toast or turn on the television, air conditioning or heating.

Finding his way around our house was also becoming increasingly difficult. He had trouble locating light switches and wardrobes also confused him. Sometimes I would find the bedroom floor littered with clean clothes and the wardrobe empty. Richard would frequently forget that wardrobes were places for keeping clothes and shoes. When the cupboard doors were shut the wardrobe became invisible to him. Once he had taken the clothes out he had no concept of returning them to the wardrobe.

One time I came home from work and went upstairs to put my briefcase away. Richard was downstairs with his late afternoon carer. I found a pot plant in our en-suite bathroom. It had been removed from its pot with the muddy roots still dangling. The loose dirt and tiny pebbles had been placed precariously over the basin drain hole. I can only guess that Richard intended to take the pot plant and plant it in a garden bed but had stopped halfway. I managed to rescue the situation by scooping dirt out with a teaspoon and picking out the tiny pebbles with a pair of tweezers thereby avoiding more unscheduled time off work and a costly visit from the plumber.

Sitting in my doctor's office one day, sleep deprived and crying uncontrollably, she delivered a stunning ultimatum to me, "Carolyn, I can't do anything to save Richard's life but I can save yours. Your life is in danger. If you don't take some time off work immediately and get some rest and look after yourself properly you are at serious risk of a heart attack, a stroke, a mental breakdown or bringing on some other form of life threatening illness."

This news hit me right between the eyes. We sat there in silence staring at each other for what seemed like an eternity but was probably only a few seconds while I processed this startling revelation. Suddenly my status had gone from being a carer to being a patient. To compound this situation, apparently I was at greater risk of dying before Richard. After that bombshell, we immediately set up regular appointments and allowed extra time for counselling.

Leaving the doctor's surgery I thought "Wow. Thanks for sugar coating the news doctor" but deep down I actually knew her ultimatum was what I really needed to hear. I can remember sobbing,

"Thank you, thank you, thank you" because finally someone had recognised the emotional pain and turmoil I was in and the impact this stress was having on me. You would think this would have been glaringly obvious to me and others around me at the time but I can see now that I was just like everyone else. I was so focussed on Richard and my children's wellbeing that I had lost sight of my own. She had given me permission to think about my own life.

On the drive home I thought of the nursery rhyme about Little Bo Peep, only instead of sheep I had lost myself and I didn't even know where to find me. It is not surprising I felt this way because Richard's prognosis due to his younger age and good health at the onset of Alzheimer's was difficult to determine. Some people with Alzheimer's can live up to twenty years but I was quickly running out of steam. For many years already I had become unconsciously engaged in the precarious, mind-bending act of trying to keep a foot in each camp. Coping with the strain of the working day and the caring night was like balancing between two different worlds and in my view it is impossible to sustain this indefinitely.

In South Australia, the Alzheimer's Association offers excellent counselling services. Unfortunately I had only managed to get to two sessions because I had taken a lot of time off work already taking Richard to doctor's appointments and other tests. I had managed to get help for Richard through the day centre and day carers at home but it never really occurred to me to ask for help for myself. I just thought I should be able to cope. I kept telling myself

I should be strong enough to look after everyone. My family was depending on me. To admit that I needed help was an untenable idea. Not so much from a sense of failure but more from fear of the potential consequences. Asking for help might suggest that cracks were appearing in my world and I was in danger of falling through one. I couldn't allow that to happen. My greatest fear was that if I crumbled we might all 'drown.'

This is one of the real dangers of carer burnout. You cannot see the wood for the trees. Like me, you may be clueless about the fact that two lives are at risk here - the person being cared for and their carer. Fortunately, I have a great doctor who rescued me before it was too late. She insisted I take sick leave from work. I was off work for nearly five months and it was during this time that arrangements were made and Richard was admitted to full time residential care. I returned to work two weeks after Richard went into care. It was a very difficult and incredibly sad time in all our lives but if left unchecked it may have even been worse.

What happens to the person with Alzheimer's if their primary carer is no longer able to look after them? Possibly the very situation that the carer is fighting to avoid in the first place may occur. Who will step up then? Who is available and capable of taking on this challenging role? The carer may be forced into relinquishing care earlier than anticipated. These are questions families and friends may want to discuss along with what they can contribute to ensure that this situation does not eventuate in their situation.

I am not going to gloss over this issue as it is one of the most important issues in this book. Readers, health insurance companies and government policy and decision makers need to understand the importance of actively supporting carers and recognise the toll that caring for Alzheimer's and other dementia sufferers takes on their carers physical and mental health. This is especially true now in light of the trend towards in-home care. I understand the economic rationale behind this policy and the popularity of deferring admission to residential care facilities. However, it is unlikely that the number of services accessible for in-home care will ever correspond with the actual need. If the primary carer burns out, undoubtedly the person they are caring for may also experience difficulties. This may result in them having to be admitted to a residential facility prematurely.

Other consequences of burnout may include the carer suffering serious or permanent illness as well as financial hardship brought about by increased medical expenses and reduced working hours. Alzheimer's Disease International research predicts that nearly fifty million people around the world are living with dementia now and that "this number will almost double every twenty years, reaching nearly seventy-five million in 2030 and over one hundred and thirty million in 2050." This explosion of dementia cases will, in turn, dramatically impact on the number of carers seeking medical services, workplace productivity, health and welfare.

TAKE-AWAYS

CHAPTER 7

It is difficult to ask for help but here are some examples to suggest to others:

- Educate yourself about the different Alzheimer's stages and behaviours so that you can better understand the type and level of stress the primary carer may be under and how you can contribute to their health and wellbeing by providing additional support

- Pick up the telephone, ask how things are going and genuinely listen

- Visit, even if it's only for ten minutes

- Contact social services on their behalf (with the carer's permission) and see what services are available and what type of assistance they might qualify for.

- When possible, include the person with Alzheimer's and their primary carer when you are entertaining, where appropriate. People still like to be asked even if they can't logistically attend.

- Do grocery shopping and help unpack and put away groceries.

TAKE-AWAYS

CHAPTER 7

- Inform and encourage extended family and friends to provide support

- Help provide transport for medical visits e.g. doctor, dentist, neurologist

- Offer to pay bills, collect dry cleaning, go to the post office.

- Put petrol in the carer's car.

- Take the carer and person with Alzheimer's out - coffee, meal or a walk.

- Come and sit with the person with Alzheimer's while their care giver goes shopping, has time to themselves or catches up with friends.

- Help clean the house, wash the dishes, do the washing or ironing.

- Tidy the garden, prune, sweep, mow.

- Put the rubbish and recycle bins out, bring in the empty bins.

TAKE-AWAYS

CHAPTER 7

- Bake a cake, make a pot of soup, cook a meal.

- Do odd jobs around the house, organise house tradesperson if required.

If you live interstate or overseas:

- Pick up the telephone, ask how things are going and listen, talk about things of interest you have been doing or a recent film, concert or event you have attended or an interesting book, magazine or article you have read.

- Organise and pay for some agency assistance (if your circumstances permit) with providing home visits, domestic chores, housekeeping, home maintenance.

- Send an email, write a nice card, send a magazine, a book or some flowers.

- Visit in person when you can.

Chapter 8

TRIGGERS - THE TIME HAS COME

Day centre, respite, residential care facility

> "It is our choices that show what we really are, far more than our abilities."
>
> *JK Rowling*

Have you ever tried driving a car while your front seat passenger is trying to climb out? It's a terrifying experience but that's exactly what happened to us on our first few trips to the dementia day centre. It didn't matter that for days I had explained to Richard multiple times the purpose of his visit to the centre or that we had been there previously to see the manager, view the facility and meet the staff. He could not remember any of that and just kept shouting, "You don't control me. You are not the boss of me. I just want to live my life." I couldn't disagree with him on that one. I probably would have said much the same thing myself if I had been in his shoes but we needed this to be a success. We had been existing with a variety of ad-hoc arrangements, utilising part-time community based support programs, extended family and friends. They were no longer a viable option. It was time to move on.

The day centre was not something that Richard warmed to immediately.

For one, all the participants were a lot older than him. Initially, he identified more with the staff because they were younger and closer to his age group and he saw them as his contemporaries. Full acceptance took a few months. He was also sensitive about the fact that he was attending a 'day centre' and I had to stop calling it that. Instead I would say, "Come on it's time to go to Norwood now," naming the suburb where the day centre was located, not the facility. That seemed to work well and over time Richard acclimatised and made friends with participants of all ages. As the centre became more familiar to him it became his sanctuary from the rest of the world and the transformation was quite noticeable. His confidence grew in such a steady, safe and secure environment. We noticed that he smiled a lot more and seemed less frustrated, bored and lonely. His life had a purpose and structure once more.

The day centre was beginning to make a difference to all of our lives. It felt like our family life had started to right itself again and tilt to a more even keel. Jack went to school, Ainslie went to university, I went to work and Richard went to Norwood. We all had somewhere to go and something to talk about at the end of the day.

Some days Richard was tired and would tend to doze off while I was cooking the dinner. This behaviour is quite common in people at the middle stage of Alzheimer's and is known as 'sun-downing,' so I kept a copy of his daily program. Sometimes he had difficulty initiating conversations but he could respond to simple questions if I asked them slowly and did not put him under any pressure to respond.

Even though Richard's days were filled with vastly different activities from when he ran a successful business, it was still very important to his confidence that he could join in and feel part of our family conversations.

Initially, Richard attended two days a week and we made alternative arrangements for the other days but this very quickly built up to Monday to Friday. The support he got from the staff and the friendship he developed with Bernie, one of the volunteers, were outstanding. The day centre provided mental stimulation, regular social interaction and an environment where activities and tasks were tailored to move at his pace, not the rest of the world's. The non-threatening surroundings helped minimise his daily frustration and assist in maintaining some level of dignity despite his diminishing abilities. Typical activities included discussion of current affairs, arts and crafts, cooking, woodwork, light gardening, card and board games, gentle exercise programs, music, concerts, excursions and picnics. There was also a barbeque in the courtyard for fine weather occasions. Richard really enjoyed doing something that was familiar to him and happily helped out with preparing the barbeque grill and with the cooking.

We all knew when Richard was at the day centre he was safe and well cared for. If he had no appetite in the evening we didn't have to worry because the staff would always give me a full report on his daily intake. The food was tasty, nutritious and plentiful with seasonal treats like hot cross buns at Easter, mince pies at Christmas and ice-creams in summer. There was fruit for morning tea, cake for afternoon tea and usually a hot meal at lunch. Some days it smelled so good when we arrived I was tempted to check myself in for the day too!

Not everyone understood why Richard needed to attend the day centre. Opinions varied enormously but we were the ones living with him and witnessing his endless struggles. Try as he would, there was just no denying that everyday activities were becoming harder and harder. Simple tasks that we all take for granted like getting dressed, combing our hair and brushing our teeth were all taking more than twice the normal time and providing a great deal of frustration and anxiety. How could zippers, buttons and shoelaces be such unfriendly and uncooperative items? Worst of all, they seemed to have a knack of misbehaving in the morning when the household was under greatest pressure.

Driving Richard to the day centre and getting to work on time was not an easy feat. Some days I would arrive at work feeling like a nervous wreck. Staff at the day centre noticed this and that our current situation was unsustainable. They advised me how to apply for partially subsidised government assistance for Richard's transportation, grooming support and supervised care. This was a huge relief and burden off our shoulders. A carer would arrive at our home in the morning and provide whatever assistance Richard needed to start his day and then drive him to the centre. In the afternoon they would pick him up and bring him home and stay with him until I got home from work.

Although this was a huge improvement to our arrangements, and I was enormously grateful, it had its flaws just like any system. There was a steady flow of strangers in our home. We had voluntarily relinquished our privacy but it took some time to adjust. Bathrobes were the order of the day if you did not want to be spotted walking down the passage in your underwear. Some days the carers turned up late and occasionally they didn't turn up at all. Rosters were changed continually so it was rare to get the same person for more than a few days or at best a week at a time. However, I firmly believe that attending the day centre enabled Richard to remain living at home for approximately five to six years longer than if the day centre and back-up support had not been available.

The day centre also acted as a conduit to access other services, including periodic residential respite care. Through talking to the staff I discovered we were eligible for sixty-three days of partially government subsidised residential respite in one year.

Jack was in the middle of Year 11 at high school. I promised him that when he was preparing for his final Year 12 exams that I would ensure he had a stress-free environment in which to study. I wasn't sure how any of us would cope. There was only one way to find out. It was time to 'put our toe in the water.' I booked Richard in for two weeks respite. This news was not well received by him. Ironically, his advancing dementia prevented him from having awareness and understanding of his diminishing abilities and there was no way he could see the need to spend time away from home and his family. We were his constant security. It was a no-win situation for me. Everything in our household revolved around supporting Richard's care but we had reached a stage where father and son had competing needs.

Young people growing up in this type of household can sometimes feel marginalised because the healthy parent is time poor, energy drained and their focus is often elsewhere. It was time to recognise Jack's needs and stand up for him. He deserved my support just as much as his father did.

As a primary carer, it is important to recognise you will never be able to please everyone. The sooner you get over the guilt and grappling with other people's expectations and lack of knowledge about Alzheimer's, the easier your life will be. You must choose your advisers carefully and listen only to them. Doctors, health care workers, case managers and professional carers all support the use of respite care. You won't have to waste time trying to convince them.

I gained this insight through Dianne, Richard's respite admission nurse. Halfway through Richard's two week respite Dianne told me an extraordinary story that put everything into perspective. I asked her how she thought Richard was settling in to the respite routine and mentioned that a few people had raised their opinion that I was doing the wrong thing. "Oh no," said Dianne, "they just have to talk to me. I could set them straight very quickly." "I heard he is having some trouble remembering which room he is sleeping in and he sometimes walks into another resident's room, ruffling a few feathers along the way." I said.

"That's pretty normal behaviour for someone with Alzheimer's, she replied "but what is really telling about Richard's level of dementia happened on the first day he arrived here. One of the staff put his suitcase on top of the bed to make it easier for him to unpack. I showed Richard his wardrobe, the en-suite bathroom, where all the light switches were and the 'call' button if he needed help. We chatted for a little while about the day centre. I assured him he could still attend even while on respite so he would not be bored or lonely. The only real difference to his routine would be that he was sleeping in the nursing home but Carolyn would be in to visit him on the weekend. He appeared to understand what I was saying and seemed quite content with those arrangements. Then I had to leave to see some of the other residents. Before I left the room I asked Richard to unpack his clothes and put them in the wardrobe and said I would be back in thirty minutes to see how he was getting along."

Tears welled in Dianne's eyes when she told me the next part of the story.

"I have seen a lot of surprising sights in my nursing career but nothing has quite prepared me for this. As I approached the room I could see the suitcase was still on the bed and all the clothes were still in it. Nothing had been touched. The wardrobe doors were wide open and there sitting inside the wardrobe on the cold hard linoleum floor was your darling husband. So you shouldn't worry too much about what other people say or think. You're the one doing the heavy lifting, not them. You and your family need this respite break.

Tell me something, are any of these people who think they know what is best for Richard volunteering to give up their own lives to look after him for respite periods or full-time?." I shook my head. "Well then, you have to look after yourself and your family. What is going to happen to Richard if you have a breakdown? He will be placed in full time residential care well before he really needs to be admitted if anything happens to you. Respite will enable Richard to live at home for as long as you are mentally and physically strong enough to continue in the carer role."

That's the day I stopped beating myself up. That's the day I got over carer guilt. I accepted that everything I did wouldn't be perfect. It is impossible to be all things to all people all the time. I couldn't be the perfect wife, mother, carer, breadwinner, friend, employee and employer. Not even close. Not even on a good day. There just weren't enough hours in the day and all those roles often seemed in competition with each other. Providing Richard with the appropriate level of daily support he needed for a clear finite period of time would have been hard enough to deal with but we couldn't even see the tunnel, let alone the light at the end of it.

The progression of Alzheimer's feels like that, relentlessly ongoing and predictably unpredictable, a seemingly never ending theft of life and spirit.

For us at home the two weeks Richard spent in respite care seemed to pass quickly. Naturally he had some challenges acclimatising to the change in routine but overall he was doing well and that was an enormous relief. Jack and I went about our usual routines of work and school but we managed to make some time for relaxation. Jack looked noticeably more at ease and he invited some friends over to the house. I was asked to join a small group of friends that were going out to dinner. I hadn't done anything like that for such a long time it felt really strange to be able to say, "Yes, count me in. I can come." I heard myself saying the words but I couldn't quite believe it was me. It wasn't just Richard who was experiencing change. We all had to learn to adjust and re-adjust.

There's a good reason why a pressure cooker releases steam slowly and that's to prevent it exploding. It wasn't until the pressure started to subside that I realised how much pressure we were really under. We had to find our way back slowly to a time when life was relatively simple and carefree in comparison.

This window into our former lives meant we didn't need convincing to try respite again and in fact we became dependent on it. Without the day centre and breaks every three to four months we would not have been able to stay together much longer as a family. Richard's total dependency on us and others around him was increasing alarmingly. More and more he needed twenty-four hour professional care.

One thing led to another and my doctor delivered an ultimatum, act now and put Richard into residential care. The other really sobering thought was that if anything happened to me and I was no longer able to care for him, he would have been placed in emergency care in a facility with which he was unfamiliar, staff he did not know and with no access to the day centre which had become his safe haven.

Faced with no alternative, I met with the director of the nursing home that was attached to the day centre.

We had discussed this transition before but it always seemed as if it was somewhere off in the distant future….something I wouldn't have to worry about just yet. Now there was no denying that the moment I had been dreading more than anything had finally arrived. There was nowhere left to hide. However, even when you have made the agonising decision to admit someone to a nursing home, it is not as simple as that. Just because you are ready doesn't mean an ideal situation will present itself to you. I had researched the admission process thoroughly and thought I was familiar with what was required but there were obstacles to overcome that I did not even know existed. During the next few weeks I felt that fortune was conspiring against us.

There had been a very recent change in the direction of aged-care policy. I believe that this was partly driven by the costs of running residential facilities which was simply becoming unsustainable. The trend was away from residential care and towards supporting people to live in their own homes longer. I was so bogged down in our everyday life that this new policy direction came as a surprise to me and very nearly defeated me at the first hurdle. When the director of the nursing home approached the chief executive of the organisation she was told quite firmly that it would not be possible to accept Richard. He did not fit the age or profile of the typical resident and would have to find alternative accommodation.

I felt as if the rug had been pulled out from beneath my feet. It was the worst possible scenario imaginable. All Richard's security was built around his family home and attending the day centre at Norwood. To put him into permanent care in unfamiliar surroundings and with people he didn't know was just not tenable. I was listening to what the director was telling me but my head was spinning. An enormous wave of shock and over-whelming failure came over me. My mission had been to keep Richard at home as long as possible and then get him into the best care available. Nothing else was acceptable. I asked her, "How do I make this right? Is there an appeal system?" "No", she replied. "I knew you would be traumatised. I have already explained to the Chief Executive (CE) that your situation is unique and I have approached him twice. I'm really so sorry but the answer is no". "There must be something I can do." Well, you could always write a letter to him outlining your case and ask him to reconsider his decision and make an exception for Richard."

Well, I thought that if I write a letter it's easier for the CE to say 'no' to a piece of paper than it will be to say 'no' to me. If I can just get an appointment and just look him in the eye, maybe I might have a chance of convincing him to make an exception. I waited a few days until I had calmed down and could think rationally. During that time I developed my strategy. Years spent working in government had taught me that the first step was to get past the 'Praetorian Guard,' also known as executive officer or executive assistant. He/

she controls the chief's appointment diary. No question that this is power in the true sense of the word. Clearly, a certain amount of due diligent planning was in order here! I wanted to know exactly who I was speaking to before I made the all important phone call. There was only going to be one shot at this and it had to be a winner.

The research paid off and after a few minutes of friendly polite conversation, I had an appointment. Phew, what a great sense of relief. But this was only the first hurdle.

There was so much hanging on the outcome of the proposed meeting that I left nothing to chance. Even what I was going to wear that day was carefully thought out. I wore my best black skirt, smart red jacket with black buttons and went to the hairdressers to have my hair blow-waved. Anything that would bring me confidence was worth doing. I also opted for corporate attire because I felt it was important to take some of the emotion out of the situation and keep the meeting on a professional level. I knew my best chance of convincing the CE to make an exception for Richard was riding on my ability to hold it together and have a calm rational discussion. Tears would not get me anywhere here.

On the morning of the meeting, after I returned from the hairdressers, I put my make-up on and donned my clothes 'ready for battle.' In my handbag, I placed an item I called my 'secret weapon,' which was ready to be pulled out if the discussion stalled.

For many years I have worked in government policy, not in law but all those years at law school would not be in vain. This was the only case I would ever truly need to win. In my mind I had rehearsed how I thought the conversation might go many times but like any negotiation there were points that were fixed and some that needed to stay fluid.

My plan was to sit at the table and keep the CE engaged long enough until he changed his mind. This wasn't going to be easy and could take some time. He kicked off with an explanation about the government policy change towards supporting elderly people to stay in their own homes longer and delaying entry into residential care because the cost of care is so expensive. I understood where this line of conversation was going and agreed that providing in-home services was good in theory provided the person being cared for had minimal needs. We chatted about this some more and then I enquired who would fill the void if there was any disconnect between the number and amount of services people were entitled to and the number and amount they actually needed.

I already knew the answer…..more and more baby-boomers would have to take on the responsibility of providing additional in-home care for their elderly parents, relatives and possibly their spouses or partners. I wondered whether they were prepared or even aware of this.

The conversation was going well so far but none of it was helping Richard. He didn't fit the usual profile of prospective nursing home residents under the old policy or the new one. As a physically fit sixty-three year old male with advanced Alzheimer's he was caught 'between a rock and a hard place' by being too young.

We were thirty-five minutes into our meeting and I was becoming increasingly nervous that the conversation was going around in circles and we were going to run out of time. Then an amazing thing happened. I noticed a little wind shift. Not exactly a breeze, more like a puff really, but it was enough to lift my spirits. We were talking more about Richard and the level of support he needed and less about the policy.

This was a good sign I thought. It was time to bring out the secret weapon.....

Ironically, I had brought it along to use if I was desperate. I had not even contemplated that it was potentially equally effective if things were going well.

Somehow I had managed to steer the conversation around to talking about Richard in the context of us as a family and the effect his illness had had on all our lives. The CE was a family man himself and appeared to be listening closely.

Then there was a slight pause in the conversation. I quickly reached into my handbag and whipped out a family photograph of Richard, myself and Ainslie and Jack taken in happier days.

It was crucial for the CE to understand this discussion wasn't just about policies and profiles. I needed to draw him into our lives. I needed to see that look I had seen on so many faces before which said, "Oh God, what if that happened to me? What if that happened to my family?" The photograph seemed the best way to illustrate the difference between whom we had been and whom we had become.

I did feel a slight twinge of shame for using such emotional blackmail but I knew I would get over it. We were a family under siege. We urgently needed his help to make an exception for Richard before something else traumatic happened. I talked about the constant stress we were all living under, the impact that was having on the children and that I had been on sick leave from work for nearly four months on my doctor's insistence.

Then there was another wind shift…..The CE mentioned a previous case of a younger person suffering from a long term illness who had been admitted and only stayed six months. This person voluntarily relocated because there was nothing wrong with their mental abilities and they said they found all the activities were not age appropriate. None of this was exactly relatable to Richard's situation but it did encourage me that there had been a precedent.

Then he mentioned Richard's relatively youthful age, his physical strength and the organisation's duty of care to protect their residents. Many of the residents had mobility and balance issues and some relied on walking frames to get around. If Richard was walking fast or not watching where he was going and happened to brush past someone frail and topple them over there was potential for serious injury. His dementia was another concern because his behaviour may be unpredictable at times. Also, the nursing home was not set up to accommodate the needs and interests of people in their early sixties. All the activities and entertainment were pitched at the eighty and ninety year olds….More Irving Berlin than Elton John….more Greta Garbo than Cate Blanchett.

I was still wondering where all this was leading when finally the CE agreed to consider Richard's situation. We had been talking for nearly an hour.

Perhaps it was the pressing argument, the secret weapon or maybe I had just exhausted him. I didn't really know and it didn't really matter. He said it would take two weeks before he would be able to get back to me with his decision. I thanked him for seeing me and his generosity with his time and promptly left his office.

When I got outside it almost came as a surprise that the sky was still blue, the traffic was still humming along and I could hear birds tweeting. I had been so focussed on the meeting that it was as if the world had ceased to exist beyond the walls of the CE's office.

I walked to the car and sat there feeling emotionally spent. I had never fought so hard for anything in my entire life. I had portrayed someone who was calm and rational despite my nerves and I believe this is what kept the CE's attention. It was the greatest acting gig of my life… my one and only 'Oscar' moment.

I hadn't got the 'yes' I was hoping for but at least there was hope.

It didn't take long before the floodgates opened. I held my face in my hands, tears poured down my cheeks and I just kept saying, "I didn't get a 'no,' I didn't get a 'no.' On reflection, I wouldn't say it was my finest hour but I had gone into battle for my family.

It was an agonising two weeks of waiting for the phone to ring and then jumping out of my skin when it did. On the fifteenth day I received my phone call from the CE. He had weighed all the facts and had not reached his decision lightly. It was a complex matter because many lives were affected by the outcome. I could tell by the tone in his voice that he was not entirely comfortable. He still had some reservations in relation to the organisation's duty of care to other residents but in the end he decided to give Richard a trial run. I would have to provide medical evidence that Richard's dementia was not of the violent/aggressive type but if I could do that then he would allow Richard to be admitted to the facility.

I thanked him sincerely and quickly got off the phone before another typhoon of tears hit. I had just been given the green light to put my husband into a nursing home. It was a strange mixture of relief and joy that Richard would be in familiar surroundings and could still visit the day centre but it was also full of deep and abiding sadness.

We got the all important letter from Richard's specialist and then the waiting began again. This wasn't like a hotel where you could ring up and make a reservation. You had to wait for the call. Every time the phone rang it sent shivers down my spine. About four weeks later I received the call from the director of the nursing home. At first I thought the offer was for a respite position. It took a few minutes to realise there was nothing temporary about the proposed arrangements. I'm not sure if that was because I was in shock or denial or a bit of both. It was just so hard to get my head around the fact that the offer was for a permanent position.

In two day's time Richard departed and never returned to our family home.

There was no question that Richard's dementia specialist, my doctor and the director of the nursing home all supported this move and said the time had definitely arrived. Richard now needed professional 24/7 care and we just couldn't provide that at home but that still didn't make it easy for us. Everything in our house revolved around Richard and his needs and without his presence there, even though the atmosphere was less stressful, the house seemed quiet and eerily empty.

Richard gradually settled in but faced some of the same challenges he did on respite, like remembering where his room was and how to find the dining room.

He still went to the day centre, although they had started scaling back his attendance times. His dementia had advanced to the extent that he now required one to one care to participate in activities and this spread the staff too thin amongst the other participants. When a vacancy came up in the secure dementia unit, it was suggested that Richard should be moved there where all the staff had more advanced training in how to cope with dementia behaviour, than staff in the general section.

This unit was actually easier for Richard because it was compact compared to the long similar looking passages in the rest of the nursing home. He could go on walks but there was no chance of getting lost and it was easier for staff to keep a constant eye on the residents.

His room was plain but functional and had a large en-suite bathroom attached. A bay window looking out onto the garden was its best feature. Before Richard moved in I dressed the room with an attractive new masculine looking bed cover, some art for the walls and a large indoor pot plant which was soon to suffer an untimely death. When the paintings were on the walls and the new pillows and cover on the bed I stood back. I had always wondered what 'the end of the road' would look and feel like and now we were there. Perhaps it was a self defence mechanism but I just felt numb all over, as if my mind was going into lock-down position and blocking out all emotions. There would be time to thaw out later after Richard was settled.

On the day of Richard's orientation into the unit one of the staff asked me to fill out some paperwork for my father! The first time that happened to me, in the doctor's office, I was quite upset but by this stage I was becoming used to it. Richard was clearly the youngest person in the unit but his dementia was accelerating the aging process and he was looking much older than someone in their early sixties.

Just like the day centre, some of the staff looked on him as a friend. They chatted to him and joked with him all the time and the level of patience, care and dedication they provided was outstanding. It can be very stressful work and it takes a very special type of person to be able to cope with that kind of pressure all the time.

It was a real bonus for Richard to have some male carers to help him shave and with other bathroom routines. Also, they would talk to him about the football or cricket which he loved. Apart from weekends when agency staff were rostered on, there was consistency in staff which was another great benefit of being in a purpose designed dementia unit.

Right before a full moon seemed to be the worst time in the unit. Nearly all the residents would become restless and difficult to handle. I found it a bit hard to believe when I first heard about this phenomenon from one of the staff but I witnessed it so many times that I became a believer. One evening I arrived just before seven in the evening. Richard was up and walking around but there was hardly anyone else sitting in the lounge area or the dining room. I asked one of the carers where everyone had gone. He told me they were nearly all in their rooms having an early night because it was the only way the staff could get them to settle down. Fortunately Richard wasn't one of the troublemakers so they were happy to assist him to get ready for bed anytime he wanted.

The decor in Richard's room was fairly sparse but this was quite intentional.

Staff advised when I was setting up Richard's room to keep to the minimalist look. Clutter of any sort can be visually distracting and confusing. Often Richard would not recognise an object because he only saw it from one angle, not in 3D. For instance, he would not recognise a drinking glass if he saw it side-on. The same thing would happen if he saw an object that was normally vertical lying in a horizontal position i.e. if he was watching me hanging some of his clothes up in the wardrobe and I asked him to pass me a coat hanger that was lying on the bench in front of him, he would just look blank and stare at me because he did not recognise the hanger when it was lying flat.

Occasionally, Richard's room was livened up by items that mysteriously appeared after he had been 'shopping.' This is common practice amongst dementia residents. They often forget where their own room is and wander in and out of each other's rooms collecting souvenirs on their travels. If they see something decorative that they fancy, the item can often be temporarily 'relocated' when they eventually find their way back to their own room.

On some visits this really made me smile. Sometimes I would pretend I was entering Aladdin's cave and wonder what exciting new treasures I would find in there. It was a case of classic recycling that did nobody any harm. There was continuity of staff so they always knew what items and photos belonged to which residents and could return them to their rightful owners. One time Richard collected a lovely pair of wooden candle sticks. The really interesting thing about this was that his taste hadn't changed even with dementia. They were just the sort of candle sticks that would have appealed to him years ago.

When Richard first went into the nursing home I was not really sure how often to visit. I was still working full time so that left mornings, evenings and weekends. In the mornings the staff were busy assisting residents with their breakfast and morning routines so this was not ideal as visitors tended to get in their way. After I finished work wasn't really suitable either because quite often by the time I got there Richard was already in bed and drifting off or fast asleep. I had a chat with the director of nursing and she suggested I get some rest during the week and reserve my visits for the weekends. This was helpful advice for many reasons.

I am not ashamed to admit that in the beginning I found it extremely confronting every time I entered the secure dementia unit. Seeing Richard in his new surroundings and how much he had deteriorated was hard enough but when other residents were having a bad day their behaviour was often affected. This was very challenging for visitors and staff.

One frail old lady used to cry out in a faint but high-pitched scream, "Help me, help me, help me," over and over again, like an LP record stuck on the needle. Staff would manage this by distracting her. Dolls the size of human babies often did the trick. Sometimes I would walk into the lounge area and think I had walked into the maternity ward by mistake. There would be a line-up of ladies nursing these life-like babies. It was amazing to see how soothing this kind of doll therapy was for them. They would cuddle the dolls and talk to them and they would burst into smiles when staff or visitors admired their little bundles of joy. Pride was written all over their faces. The effect could not have been greater if they had been real babies.

Music was another tool for settling down agitated residents. It was often played over the public address system throughout the unit.

Andre Rieu's concert video was a popular feature in the lounge room. Lively classical and waltz music combined with elaborate colourful costumes attracted a regular fan base. It was pure 'feel good' entertainment with no complicated or confusing plots to frustrate this particular audience. Residents could just sit back and enjoy or sing along if they felt so inclined….and they often did.

Some residents needed more help than others. Richard was one of these. Even though he was the youngest person in the unit he often needed individual help. After Richard had been in there about three years his weight suddenly crashed. At first no one could work out why, until an observant carer who looked after him on a regular basis said they thought Richard might have forgotten how to feed himself because he was leaving a lot of food on his plate and making little attempt to eat. Sure enough, once a staff member was assigned to sit with him and spoon feed him all his meals every day his weight returned and he recovered his interest in food although he never regained the ability to feed himself again.

I visited every weekend. Sometimes I would time my visit for late Saturday afternoon and stay and feed him his dinner. Memories of us as young parents, spoon feeding Ainslie and Jack when they were babies would flash in my mind and now I was spoon feeding their father. I found this really tough but Richard often did not know the weekend staff as well so it helped if I was there to feed him. It was also another way of spending time with him when he was no longer able to engage in conversation because he was losing the ability to construct sentences.

Every now and then one of the younger more agile ladies would join us if we were walking in the garden. This lady would be perfectly fine until her daughter arrived and then she would burst into tears and sob the whole time she was there. After she left the tears would stop and the staff would find something to distract her with until she smiled again.

Another gentleman asked for my help to telephone his daughter to come and pick him up because he couldn't stay there any longer. He said he needed to get home urgently because he was running late and his wife would be wondering where he was. I spoke to one of the nurses and she told me he often said that but the problem was that his wife had died six years before.

Richard lived in the nursing home for five years and his last four were spent in the dementia unit. I visited him every weekend except for a few short holidays and our children visited when they could. The unit provided Richard with a level of care that was simply outstanding and way beyond any physical capabilities of one person functioning alone. As Alzheimer's ravaged his memory, his everyday needs increased exponentially. Providing support to get in and out of bed, bathing, feeding, dressing and coping with incontinence for someone with severe memory loss is hugely demanding. These routine daily tasks were outsourced for Richard but not our care or love. The tragic circumstances that required him to live under a different roof in a different location could never drive him from our hearts.

For the majority of years that Richard was in the nursing home neither Ainslie nor Jack lived in the family home. Ainslie moved to London and Jack lived in Queensland and then the Northern Territory. Yes, we were spread far and wide. It was by no means ideal but geography did not diminish our feelings. There are invisible chains of love that link us all together no matter where we live, whether it's overseas, interstate or even in a nursing home just a fifteen minute drive across town.

TAKE-AWAYS

CHAPTER 8

- This disease runs its own race, with its own timetable

- You have to make long term plans but be ready to make adjustments - constantly tweak them

- Keep everything fluid - like wet cement

- A dementia day centre can impact positively on everyone in the family

- It is important to recognise the needs of all members in the family

- Sometimes other members of the family will have more pressing needs than the person with Alzheimer's

- You cannot please everyone so listen to advice selectively

- Other people's expectations and lack of knowledge about Alzheimer's is not your concern

- Listen to the medical professionals and learn to get over carer's guilt

TAKE-AWAYS

CHAPTER 8

- You may have to persevere to get a place in the nursing home of your choice

- Placing someone in a nursing home does not mean you have abandoned them

- Love is not diminished by geography

Chapter 9

FINDING RESILIENCE

Adapting to stress and adversity

> "It is not the strongest of the species that survives but the most adaptable."
>
> *Attributed to Charles Darwin*

It was early 2014 and I was visiting Richard in the garden attached to the secure dementia unit where he had been living for the last four years. We were sitting on a wooden bench located next to the make-believe yellow and black bus stop which looks exactly like the real thing. The bus stop is there for the benefit of recently admitted residents who are still settling into life in the unit. Some residents who have not quite adjusted to their new surroundings often ask nursing staff if they can 'go home' to visit their spouse or partner, even though their spouse or partner may have been dead for many years. Sometimes the kindest way to handle this kind of loss is with distraction. Sitting at the bus stop happily waiting for a bus that is never coming is far less emotionally stressful than the jolt received when told that your loved one has been dead for years. I have seen many looks of fear, anguish and deep confusion when 'helpful' visitors and family members have pointed out to residents that their loved ones are no longer "with us." I believe that it is far better to sit in a lovely peaceful garden and forget why you came outside in the first place.

On this particular Saturday there were no other 'travellers' on the bench. I could see Richard was revelling in the fresh air with the warmth of the sun on his face. He was a country boy born and bred and so he loved being surrounded by all the flowers, shrubs and trees. He was spending most of his time inside by then and he looked like he really enjoyed the freedom of being outdoors and the joy of gazing up at a brilliant blue sky through the gum tree canopy.

Richard had long since lost the art of conversation and when he did attempt speech the words came out garbled and barely recognisable more often than not. Often I would take a newspaper or magazine for our visits and read out stories about sport and current affairs that in the past he would have been interested in. Other residents enjoyed this too. It wasn't long before I developed a bit of a fan club. 'Click-clack' went the sound of the walking frames on linoleum and I knew my followers were on their way! They would gather around or even come and sit at our table and listen to the latest news items and human interest stories. I liked the real estate and travel pages best so they probably got an unhealthy overdose of marketplace activity reports and endless tips on how to snare luxury cruise deals for bargain basement prices but they didn't seem to mind and certainly never complained.

Unlike Richard, the majority of the 'fan club' had mobility issues, so when the staff were busy providing toileting assistance or preparing the dining room they were temporarily anchored in front of the television and prevented from joining us outside. That was the case this particular afternoon, so we had the whole garden to ourselves. We just sat there peacefully basking in the sun, taking in all the scenery and drinking our coffee in silence. It was forty-five minutes into the visit when the 'ambush' happened. It came out of nowhere. I had been prepping myself for years but still I never saw it coming.

I was looking at Richard and smiling at him and he smiled back at me. Then this puzzled look came across his face. He looked at me directly in the eyes and said in quite clear speech that anyone could have understood, "Who are you? Do I know you?"

I was so totally taken by surprise. The words just seemed to freeze in the air. My mind went straight into overdrive, spinning in every direction. I knew I had only a few seconds to decide what my response would be. Whatever I said would take Richard a few moments to process even if he could understand what I said. Buying time, I plastered a big smile on my face.

So having come all this way, after facing all of the challenges, here we were again years later. It felt as if we were back at the beginning. I had to make a decision: victim or survivor, what was it going to be?

Instinctively, I reached out and put my arm around Richard and said, "Oh yes, we go back a long way. We have been friends for years."

I didn't say another word. I knew Richard would have struggled to digest any more information than that but also I was unable to say anything else. My eyes had watered up. Somehow I managed to keep smiling. Richard smiled back. He seemed to be happy with my response, obviously pleased to work out a connection. Then just as quickly for him the moment was gone forever.

Behind the smile, I was in a state of emotional shock. Although I had been mentally preparing myself for years the reality was far more confronting and harder to cope with than I had rehearsed all those times.

I picked up our coffee cups and took Richard by the arm and walked him around the garden a few more times while I processed what had just happened.

We did several loops before it hit me that Richard had just constructed and articulated two perfect sentences and each in context with the other. This was an astonishing effort for him in his advanced stage of Alzheimer's. I hadn't heard him talk that clearly in years. The fact that he didn't know me shouldn't diminish his accomplishment. I always knew the day would come when this would happen and so now it had finally arrived. I could let it take me under or I could celebrate Richard's two sentences. I decided to run with the latter option. Besides, if I had let myself go, Richard would not have been able to work out why I was upset; only that something was wrong. He had enjoyed the visit. That was as good a result as I could hope for. "Best leave it at that," I thought. "I'll deal with my emotions later when they are not quite so raw."

By this time the sun was losing its warmth so we went inside and I got Richard settled in an armchair and then told Julie, one of Richard's nurses what had happened. She looked at me with a grin that said to me, "...and you are pleased about that?" I felt suddenly foolish. But then broke into a full smile and said, "Actually, when you think about it, that's pretty amazing for Richard isn't it?"

Julie had been looking after Richard for a few years by then. She knew how much his speech had deteriorated and so we agreed it was better to focus on his achievement not his actual words. After all, Richard and I had come such a long way from when he was diagnosed that this was just another milestone along the Alzheimer's highway.

Nevertheless, I was still shaking and teary eyed when I left the unit and I could barely remember the security code to get out of there but as I walked through the door and looked down the long empty passage, I felt some of the weight on my shoulders ease slightly. As I drove out of the car park, tears were still streaming down my cheeks but I gulped another big sigh of relief and slowly accelerated towards the world where I belonged.

Fortunately, I had grocery shopping to do after the visit. I found it quite comforting standing in the check-out aisle with a big queue in front of me. Such a common everyday scene brought me back to reality with a thud. Somewhere between the trolleys filled with fruit and vegetables, weekend sales items and other household essentials some measure of resilience kicked in. While I was waiting to be served I just kept repeating to myself over and over, "It's only words, it's only words." Richard's dementia was so advanced he could just as easily have said those words to one of the staff or any of the other residents.

The real world was calling me back. I could feel it and I was only too glad to answer. That evening I had plans to go out to dinner with good friends Jill and Tony, at our favourite Thai restaurant. There was time just enough to unpack the groceries, repair my blotchy face, change my clothes and arrive at the restaurant at 7:15pm. How wonderful to be greeted by warm friendly faces and talk about normal things. Jill asked about my day so I told them but somewhere between the Pad Thai noodles and the red chicken curry we decided not to dwell on it. We reminisced about holidays we had enjoyed together and it was the best medicine in the world! I couldn't stay sad all the time and I know that would have been the last thing Richard would have wanted.

It wasn't until a few days later when I had had some space that I had the opportunity to process what had actually happened. I realised that I had finally arrived at a significant survival point. The moment I had been dreading for years, when Richard didn't know me, had come and gone. The world hadn't ended. Our lives continued. Nothing was the same as before but I knew I had developed a certain degree of resilience.

TAKE-AWAYS

CHAPTER 9

- Reading out loud is a great way to spend time visiting with someone who has trouble communicating with you

- Take your favourite newspaper or magazine and read that out loud and then you can both benefit

- Even if someone can't understand what you are saying they can always understand a smile

- Even two sentences are worth celebrating

- Sometimes emotions require some time and space to absorb

- Routine chores can be quite comforting at times because they can bring a sense of normality to a stressful situation

- Carers need to spend time with people who are not under similar stress

- Even an event you have prepared yourself for many times can still take you by surprise

Chapter 10

THE TRILOGY OF GRIEF

Before, during, after

> "And where does the power come from,
> to see the race to its end? From within."
>
> *Eric Liddell, quoted in the movie "Chariots of Fire"*

To many of the congregation gathered at Richard's funeral, news of his death may have come as a shock but for those who stayed close, his death had been a long time coming. Richard lived approximately eighteen years from when the signs of memory loss first started to appear.

In South Australia a person is officially considered an adult when they reach eighteen years of age. They can vote, fight for their country, drink alcohol in public places and enter legally binding contracts. No wonder Richard's illness felt like it had lasted a lifetime – because indeed it actually had.

Prior to Richard's death, I had experienced intense grief when my father and later my mother died of age related illnesses. I found their deaths were both extremely painful at the time but I understood their passing as part of the cycle of life. Funeral services were held to celebrate lives well lived and close family, friends and relatives all came together to pay their respects and honour their memory. This is the normal experience that most people encounter – first the death, then the grieving, then for those left behind, a period of adjustment and then moving on.

This is often referred to as the Stages of Grieving. The origins are Elisabeth Kubler-Ross' book, *On Death and Dying* which explains the stages of the feelings and emotions involved in the grieving process: Denial, Anger, Bargaining, Depression and Acceptance.

However, when someone you love has dementia the primary caregiver and immediate family and friends experience all that and more. They get to grieve three times. The first period of grief you encounter is at the time of diagnosis. The second is while living with dementia and the third is at the end of life when you grieve afresh....all over again.

The second period of grief is, in my experience, the most difficult of all. Due to the slow nature of Alzheimer's, the grief experienced by family and friends is relentless. There is nothing you can do to resolve it, except learn to live each day floating in a cocktail of emotions and runaway feelings. Throughout the course of the disease the carers watch their loved one slip away day by day. This concept of unresolved grief is best explained by Dr Pauline Boss in her wonderfully enlightening book, *Ambiguous Loss*. I wish I had discovered it earlier. Unfortunately, Richard's decline was well advanced when I read this book but I thoroughly recommend it to anyone looking for this type of advice.

I think most people who have experienced some form of grief will agree that processing grief takes time. You can't rush it or fast forward it and you can't control it. Grief washes over you in waves. It hits you when you least expect it.

You can be fine one minute and then something unexpected happens that triggers a memory. Suddenly you see, hear, smell and taste or experience something that transports you back in time and place faster than a 'Delorean time machine'.

There is no timeline with grief. It is an entirely personal thing. Everyone has their own pace and no one should ever feel pressured to rush it just because the rest of the world has moved on. It does take time to work through but it doesn't have to last forever. I believe that sometimes people hold on to grief because they can't imagine the alternative, as if continuing the grieving process keeps the memory of their loved one alive, but there is an alternative way to look at this. Perhaps the best way to release yourself from grief is to honour the dead by going on and leading a full, rich and rewarding life. It has really helped me to focus on what Richard would have wanted, not on feeling sad, lonely and sorry for us.

It is not just losing your partner to Alzheimer's and the impact this has on you that you grieve for but for the loss of your way of life and the joint dreams and plans that will now go unrealised, such as sharing retirement and the possibility of grandchildren.

One night, after Richard had gone into care and Ainslie and Jack had left home, the burglar alarm in our house went off at 3am. This gave me a terrible scare because I was unaware that it was armed. (We had stopped using it years before when Richard could not remember the code.) The next day the security experts advised that it was possibly a spider crawling over the sensor that had triggered the alarm but it gave me such a fright that it shocked me into thinking about my own life and where, if anywhere, it was going.

I understood only too well that there was nothing I could do to change Richard's life but I could change my own. What was the point of living in a family sized home on my own? Just a lot of empty walls that never talked back.

Moving out of the house would give me a fresh start and help ease the stress of living every day surrounded by memories of the past and with no vision of the future. I had come to the conclusion that a life lived permanently on hold is no life at all.

I had lived in an empty house for over two years. Now it was time for action!

A small but cosy one bedroom apartment nearby became vacant, so I rented out the family home and booked the removalist company. It was a hefty dose of self-imposed tough love but at least I had found a way to move on.

Although it would be a welcome relief not to have to walk down the hallway past closed doors leading to empty rooms, moving out was still not easy. Decades of accumulated furniture and belongings had to be sorted and memories had to be "filed away" to be dealt with at a later date. It had taken over thirty years to put this life together and I dismantled it in three days.

As I walked past packing boxes and cases and through room after empty room tears flowed freely down my dusty cheeks. It wasn't another typical Maybelline day for me, it was a Maybelline marathon, but I knew it had to be done.

Looking back now, it was one of the best things I did towards reclaiming my life. Two years alone in the house was long enough. However, this 'waiting period' had given me the necessary time to process my thoughts and to start accepting the fact that the 'nest' was empty and I was truly on my own. The house without the family's presence no longer felt like a home. I still admired some of the architectural features such as the fireplace, ornate ceilings and traditional leadlight windows but I came to recognise it was all just timber, bricks and mortar, steel and glass. It had sheltered my body but not my soul. Unlike my family, there was nothing there that was irreplaceable, nothing that I couldn't live without or leave behind.

As I walked out of the front door for the last time, I thanked the wandering spider who had frightened me into action and pushed me nervously towards a new life. Ironically, the apartment I had found was only two streets away from the home we purchased when we were first married and before the children were born. It felt as if my life was turning full circle. It was certainly a different life than what I had dreamed of back then but at least the long feelings of paralysis were fading. I had given myself permission for my life to move on.

TAKE-AWAYS

CHAPTER 10

- Look back and treasure the relationship you once had

- Families loving someone with Alzheimer's and other types of dementia get to grieve three times, before, during and after

- Grieving is an entirely personal process and different for everyone

- Grief doesn't have to last forever

- Alzheimer's can last so long and be so destructive that grieving starts before the death

- Carers sometimes need to move on with their own lives as a means of surviving continuous grieving

THE ENDING

In my experience, 'the end' is never quite how you expect it to be even when you think you are prepared and you know it is coming. Death somehow still manages to sneak up and then shock all those who look upon the dying with a sense of certainty. For most of us, it is impossible to grasp this until the moment finally arrives.

We had twelve years after the diagnosis to prepare for Richard's death yet still it came as a surprise. There were so many false alarms along the way including a near-fatal heart attack and many significant seizures and falls that my sense of the inevitable had diminished considerably when the end finally came.

Over the years, I was frequently amazed at Richard's physical ability to bounce back from every setback. I began to think he had morphed himself into a hybrid of the biblical figure Lazarus and the great magician Houdini.

Eventually however, the great release that is death came calling and Richard had reached his elastic limit. He had no bounces left to give. Even so, he was still a reluctant traveller and struggled for nearly a week before embracing the final surrender.

Signs of Richard's final decline were first noticed by the nursing staff but the significance of their comments initially escaped me. Given Richard's past history of false alarms, the fact that he was having an afternoon nap in bed when I came to visit didn't particularly disturb me. It was only when I discovered that he was becoming more reluctant to get out of bed each morning without considerable coaxing by staff that I realised he was unlikely to recover this time. When I fully understood the significance of the events that were about to unfold, I sat by Richard's bed every day, holding his hand, soothing his brow, talking to him, telling him happy stories to send him on his way with our blessings.

At the time, Ainslie was married and living in London and Jack was working in Darwin. I kept them informed of events as they transpired. We talked about whether they should rush home or wait till they heard from me. The last time Ainslie saw her father was seven and a half months earlier on the day before her wedding. It nearly broke her heart when her Dad did not recognise her. "I would rather remember Dad as he was before he became ill," she said. Jack visited Richard whenever he was in Adelaide. He knew what it felt like too and he also decided to wait for the news. I told them it was entirely their choice. Richard, as always unselfish, would not have wanted it any other way.

Palliative care of the dying is a gift of self that is not for the faint hearted. However, during this sad and difficult time I was blessed in having three very special friends, Jill, Anne and Lindy, who volunteered to help me and took it in shifts to sit at Richard's bedside with me or sat with him whilst another ensured I took a breather from my bedside vigil and had something to eat and drink.

Watching Richard's chest rise and fall and then listening to him going through the 'death rattle' was excruciating for everyone but their love, courage, loyalty and support for us never faltered.

As each day ended the overwhelming tiredness and emotional toll was evident on their faces but it was crystal clear to me that their thoughts were only about what they could give in support, not what the experience was taking out of them. I have never witnessed or experienced such unselfish friendship before in my life. It was friendship in its truest form – pure gold and strong as diamonds.

When Ainslie moved to London I missed her enormously but I wanted her to live the life she would have lived if her father had not become ill. I knew with absolute certainty that he would have wanted that more than anything too. Ainslie has made wonderful progress in her career and she and her husband Tom are very happy enjoying life and all the opportunities London has to offer. Jack has resigned from his job and returned to university in Queensland to finish his degree. I am so proud of both my children. Their father would have been too. They have both come through balanced and happy and without 'a chip on their shoulder' and are making a success of their lives. I believe Richard's memory is honoured by the lives that they are leading - a fitting testimony to one of nature's true gentlemen.

AUTHOR PROFILE

Carolyn Cranwell

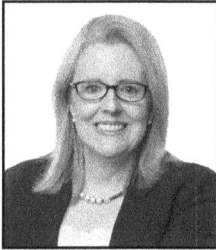

Carolyn is an author, lawyer and senior transport security advisor for government and a former dental nurse and hygienist. She has had eighteen years experience as an Alzheimer's carer. Carolyn is determined to raise awareness of the challenges and impact that long-term Alzheimer's caring has on families and to lessen the stigma associated with this disease in Australia and beyond.

At the age of twenty two Carolyn returned to study and attended the University of Adelaide Law School. She married her husband Richard in March 1982. Combining study, work and raising her family, she completed her law degree (LLB) before going on to earn her Graduate Diploma in Legal Practice (GDLP). After graduating, she spent fifteen years working in various public service roles including providing advice to State Government Ministers and Executives on counter-terrorism and emergency management for the public transport system. Carolyn was widowed in November 2014.

Carolyn loves reading, property renovation and design, travel and walking through the parklands in her home city of Adelaide. As a child she loved to sit on her grandmother's knee gazing at souvenir travel books and hearing tales of sailing to England, Scotland and beyond via the Suez Canal. She has travelled to England, Europe, New Zealand, the United States, Canada, Singapore, Vietnam, Laos, Hong Kong, India, the United Arab Emirates, Denmark, Greece, Tunisia, Ireland, Portugal, France, Monte Carlo, Spain, Italy and throughout Australia.

Carolyn Cranwell is the author of 'Navigating Alzheimer's' and lives near the inner city in Adelaide, South Australia. She has two adult children, Ainslie and Jack and a son-in-law Tom.

RESOURCES

Where can I find more information about Alzheimer's disease?

In Australia the **Alzheimer's Australia** website (**www. fightdementia.org.au**) provides information about memory loss, including advice that may help you to distinguish between normal memory loss and memory loss associated with dementia.

United Kingdom
(**www.alzheimer's .org.uk/**)

USA
(**www.alz.org/**)

Alzheimer's Disease International (ADI) (**www.alz.co.uk/**)
ADI is the worldwide federation of Alzheimer's associations, which supports people with dementia and their families.

Where can I get more information about Support Services?

National Dementia Helpline

In Australia you can call the National Dementia Helpline on **1800 100 500** for information.

The Australian government offers a range of services for Australian citizens that may enable an older person to stay in their own home longer by accessing a Home Care Package.

A **Home Care Package** may provide:
- Support services for domestic help
- Personal care
- Nursing, allied health and clinical services
- Care coordination and case management

For information on **Residential Aged Care Homes:**
Website (**www.myagedcare.gov.au**)

OTHER RESOURCES

Chris Christoff

Author of "Goal Setting for People Who Can't Set Goals - Proven Tools and Techniques to Achieve Anything You Want"

www.YouCanSetGoals.com

McInerney Barratt - Financial Solutions

Aged Care is a specialised area of Financial Planning
"McInerney Barratt Financial Solutions, through their close relationship with the aged care industry and their financial planning experience in this area, have become the financial advisers of choice to the aged care industry."

www.mbfs.com.au/

FREQUENTLY ASKED QUESTIONS

What is Dementia?

Understanding dementia can be confusing because it is a condition rather than a disease. This condition is a collection of symptoms that can be caused by various diseases.

Dementia causes ongoing gradual deterioration of the brain and is a terminal illness. Common symptoms that are associated with decline of the brain and its abilities may include impaired:

- Memory
- Thinking
- Language
- Understanding
- Judgement

There are many types and causes of dementia including Alzheimer's disease, injury to the brain, stroke or other diseases such as Huntington's Lewy body Dementia, Parkinson's and Cruezfeldt-Jakob disease.

NAVIGATING ALZHEIMER'S

What is Alzheimer's Disease?

Alzheimer's disease is the most common form of dementia. It accounts for between 50% and 70% of all types of dementia. Alzheimer's disease is a degenerative condition that affects the brain. As brain cells die, the substance of the brain shrinks causing certain information to no longer be recalled or understood. (www. myagedcare.gov.au)

Alzheimer's is most common in people aged 65 years or over but can occur in people much younger. This may be known as Early Onset or Younger Onset Alzheimer's. There is currently no cure available for Alzheimer's but there are some drugs that may help symptoms in the early stages of the disease.

What are the Top Ten Early Warning Signs for dementia?

The early warning signs include subtle changes including:
- Short term memory loss - (forgetting items like keys, dates and names)
- Communication difficulties - (struggling to find the right words)
- Confusion - (forgetting time and familiar places)
- Changes in mood - (behaviour and personality changes)
- Distraction - (difficulty in performing routine tasks)
- Social withdrawal - (loss of interest and confidence in social interaction)

- Vision and spatial skills decline - (loss of sense of direction)
- Decline in abstract thinking - (difficulty balancing a cheque book)
- Loss of initiative - (waits for direction before taking action)
- Struggles with change - (new tasks, routines, places)

What is an MMSE test?

This test is usually conducted by a doctor or specialist in their office and takes around 5 minutes to complete. The MMSE is the most common test for the screening of dementia. It assesses skills such as reading, writing, orientation and short-term memory. (www.fightdementia.org.au)

What is a Computed Tomography (CT) scan?

This is an imaging procedure that uses x-rays and digital computer technology to create detailed pictures of the body. It can image every type of body structure at once, including blood vessels, bone and soft tissue. (www.betterhealth.vic.gov.au)

What is Magnetic Resonance Imaging (MRI)?

This technique uses powerful magnets and microwaves to produce very clear 3-dimensional images of the brain. As well as ruling out treatable causes of dementia, MRI can reveal patterns of brain tissue loss, which can be used to discriminate between different forms of dementia such as Alzheimer's disease and frontotemporal dementia.
(www.fightdementia.org.au)

What is a dementia day centre?

A dementia day centre offers people with dementia an opportunity to participate in a broad range of interesting activities and social gatherings in a safe, supportive, caring, understanding and non-threatening environment. Regular communication, companionship and a sense of purpose are some of the key benefits for participants attending a dementia day centre.

What is respite care?

Respite care is a form of support for the person with dementia and the carer. It gives the carer an opportunity to catch up on everyday activities and to rest. This might mean going on a holiday or just recuperating at home knowing that the person they care for and all their daily needs are being attended to by trained staff at a residential facility or possibly by family or a friend.

In Australia, for information about respite care and services:
Telephone the **My Aged Care** contact centre on **1800 200 422**
Website **www.myagedcare.gov.au**

What is palliative care?

The aim of palliative care is to achieve the best possible quality of life for the person with a life-limiting illness and provide support for their family and carers.

Palliative care:
- Affirms life and treats dying as a normal process
- Neither hastens or delays death
- Provides relief from pain and other distressing symptoms
- Integrates the physical, psychological, social, emotional and spiritual aspects of care, with coordinated assessment and management of each person's needs

- Offers support to help people live as actively as possible until death
- Offers support to help the family during the person's illness and in their own bereavement

www.ingramcontent.com/pod-product-compliance
Lightning Source LLC
Chambersburg PA
CBHW072237270326
41930CB00010B/2166